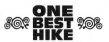

ONE BEST HIKE

MT. WHITNEY

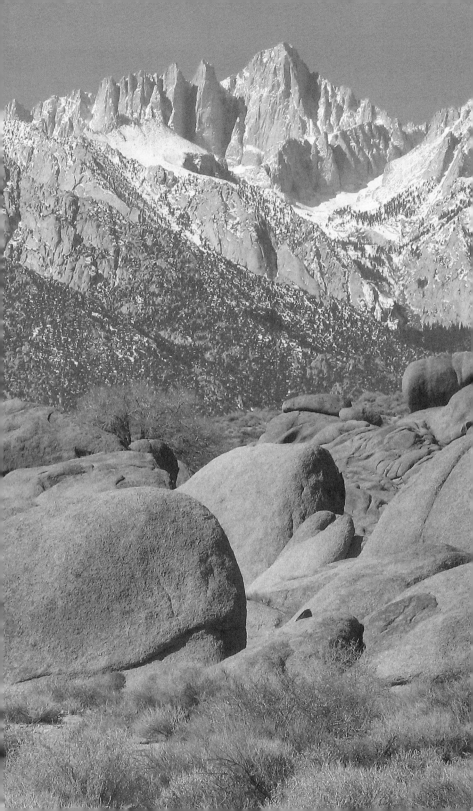

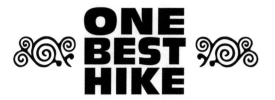

MT. WHITNEY

Everything you need to know to successfully hike California's highest peak

Elizabeth Wenk

 WILDERNESS PRESS ... *on the trail since 1967*

One Best Hike: Mt. Whitney

1st EDITION September 2008
  2nd printing 2011

Copyright © 2008 by Elizabeth Wenk

Cover photos copyright © 2008 by Elizabeth Wenk
Interior photos, except where noted, © 2008 by Elizabeth Wenk

Cover design: Larry B. Van Dyke
Book design: Andreas Schueller and Larry B. Van Dyke

ISBN 978-0-89997-464-4

Manufactured in the United States of America

Published by: **Wilderness Press**
        Keen Communications
        PO Box 43673
        Birmingham, AL 35243
        (800) 443-7227; FAX (205) 326-1012
        info@wildernesspress.com
        www.wildernesspress.com

Visit our website for a complete listing of our books and for ordering information.

Distributed by Publishers Group West

Front cover photos: Top: Mt. Whitney as seen from the Whitney Portal Road;
  Middle: The Smithsonian Instiution summit shelter; *Bottom:* Hiking up the 99
  switchbacks, through a section blasted into a cliff face
Back cover photos: Top: A pinnacle near Trail Crest; *Bottom:* Trail Camp is a beauti-
  ful high-elevation campsite
Frontispiece: Mt. Whitney viewed from the Whitney Portal Road in the Alabama
  Hills

SAFETY NOTICE: Although Wilderness Press and the author have made every attempt to ensure that the information in this book is accurate at press time, they are
not responsible for any loss, damage, injury, or inconvenience that may occur to
anyone while using this book. You are responsible for your own safety and health
while in the wilderness. The fact that a trail is described in this book does not mean
that it will be safe for you. Be aware that trail conditions can change from day to
day. Always check local conditions and know your own limitations.

Acknowledgements

I dedicate this book to all who have showed me the many ways that mountains, especially those in the Sierra Nevada, can be endlessly captivating and enchanting.

I thank my husband, Douglas, for his support while I wrote this book. And I thank my young daughter, Eleanor, for being tolerant of many hours sitting in a backpack. While I photographed mountains on a decidedly chilly November afternoon, she appropriately took her first backcountry steps at Trail Camp.

Carolyn Tiernan, M.D., carefully reviewed all medical sections, providing important feedback. Hal Klieforth commented on the text on Sierra weather and human history and provided me unlimited access to his extensive library of Sierra literature.

I add my appreciation to Wilderness Press for providing me the opportunity to write this book. They allowed me the freedom to express my approach to hiking: that you need to look at and think about natural history and human history as you follow the trail upwards.

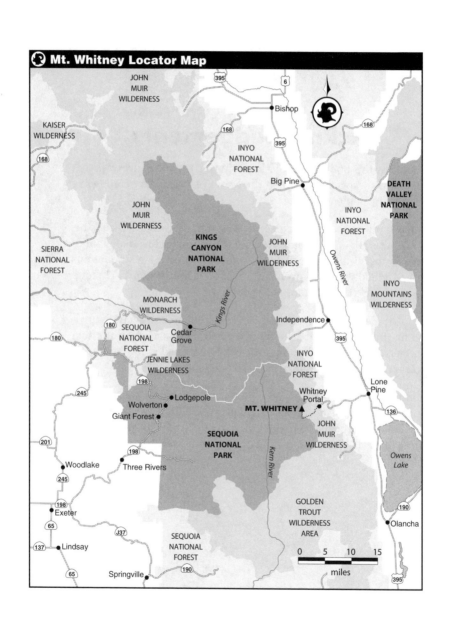

Mt. Whitney Locator Map

JOHN MUIR WILDERNESS

KAISER WILDERNESS

168

395

6

Bishop

168

168

395

INYO NATIONAL FOREST

Big Pine

DEATH VALLEY NATIONAL PARK

JOHN MUIR WILDERNESS

KINGS CANYON NATIONAL PARK

JOHN MUIR WILDERNESS

INYO NATIONAL FOREST

Owens River

SIERRA NATIONAL FOREST

MONARCH WILDERNESS

Kings River

INYO MOUNTAINS WILDERNESS

180

SEQUOIA NATIONAL FOREST

Cedar Grove

Independence

395

180

JENNIE LAKES WILDERNESS

INYO NATIONAL FOREST

198

Whitney Portal

Lone Pine

245

Lodgepole

MT. WHITNEY ▲

136

Wolverton

Giant Forest

JOHN MUIR WILDERNESS

201

SEQUOIA NATIONAL PARK

Owens Lake

198

Woodlake

Three Rivers

Kern River

245

198

Exeter

GOLDEN TROUT WILDERNESS AREA

190

65

J37

Olancha

137

Lindsay

SEQUOIA NATIONAL FOREST

0   5   10   15

65

Springville

190

miles

395

Contents

Right: Enjoying a breather and snack beside pinnacles at Trail Crest

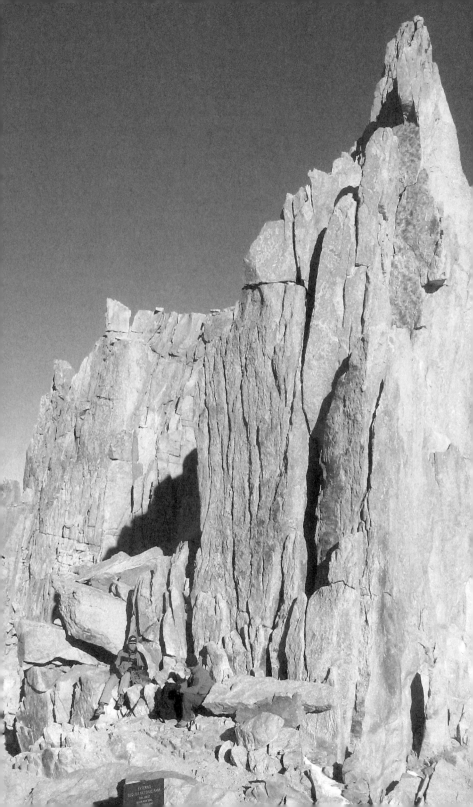

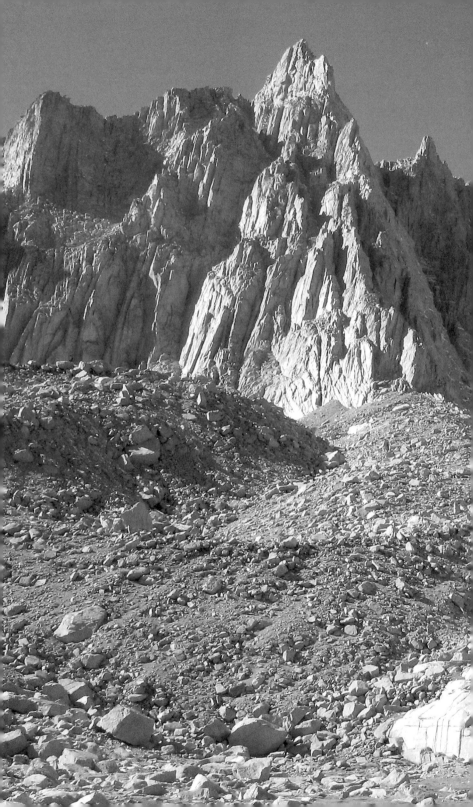

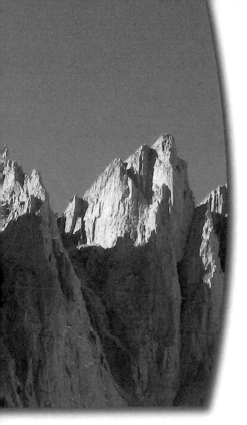

1
Introduction

Whitney is easily accessible to all whose heart and lungs can stand its rarified atmosphere, and probably no other mountain in the world unascended by a railway can boast such an enrollment of visitors.

—Marion Parsons,
the first woman to serve on the Sierra Club board of directors, and a member of a 1909 Sierra Club ascent of Mt. Whitney

Mt. Whitney and the Mt. Whitney Trail

The summit of Mt. Whitney has been a sought-after point ever since 1864, when the peak was first surveyed as the highest in the United States. Although the number of ascents per year has risen hundredfold since Parsons' time, her sentiments still ring true today. One of the most iconic peaks in the country, 14,505-foot Whitney stands 72 feet higher than Colorado's Mt. Elbert, making it the highest peak in the contiguous 48 states (Alaska's 20,320-foot Denali is the highest in the United States).

Mt. Whitney's top is a desired destination for reasons other than its lofty elevation: It's a beautiful peak, in easy driving reach of 30 million people, and the challenging but non-technical trail makes reaching the summit an attainable goal for almost anyone in good shape. The steep, eastern face of Mt. Whitney is exquisite—the last in a dramatic series of jagged peaks, nearly each one higher than the previous, culminating in the summit of Mt. Whitney. This vista is powerful from the peak's base town of Lone Pine, 10,000 feet below in the Owens Valley.

Opposite and above: The Whitney crest, in the vicinity of Mt. Muir, as seen from Trail Camp

Perhaps most important, the summit is not a giveaway. Whitney is tough enough to give you a real challenge, but not so tough that you need technical mountaineering equipment and a guide. Indeed, the 21-mile trail (up and back) is a distance most people can hike with appropriate training and planning.

It is the Mt. Whitney Trail that makes the summit an achievable goal. Before the trail was built, in 1904, it was impossible to summit in a day or even a long weekend, as Hubert Dyer, an early Sierra mountaineer and a charter member of the Sierra Club, reported in 1893:

> *To one standing near these structures, the stupendous mass of the Sierras seems hanging over them, and the summit of Whitney but a little way off. Yet it is about 70 miles by the shortest trail to the summit. There are stories told of men who have climbed the great eastern face. Though possible, it is a dangerous undertaking.*

Today, about 10,000 people each year successfully reach the top of Mt. Whitney by the easiest route to the summit, the well-maintained, 10.5-mile Mt. Whitney Trail, which ascends one route up that "great eastern face." There's no reason why you can't be one of them.

The goals of this book are threefold. First, it aims to provide novice hikers and hikers new to the high-elevation Sierra Nevada with the background information to safely summit Mt. Whitney—or to

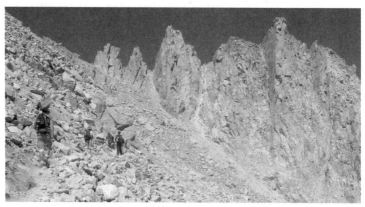

The final switchback before Trail Crest

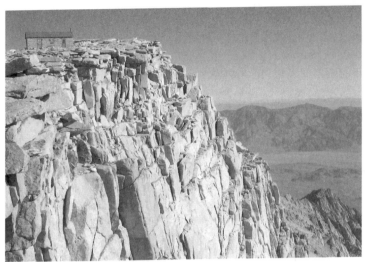

Mt. Whitney's summit and the Smithsonian Institution research hut

know when conditions such as health or weather mean it's time to turn around and make another summit bid in the future. It is also meant to provide the information all hikers need to plan a summit bid: details on wilderness permits, what to eat and where to sleep in Lone Pine, what gear is essential, and, of course, everything you need to know about hiking up the Mt. Whitney Trail itself. This book will also give you a better understanding of the human and natural history of the Mt. Whitney area.

Many people, especially dayhikers, will rightfully question the notion of carrying a guidebook to the summit of the peak. When will you have time to admire plants or geologic features on the ascent? My advice is to read the sections "Precautions and Considerations" (page 33) and "Preparations and Planning" (page 51) before your hike. Then photocopy the route description, elevation profile, sketch map of the route, and the labeled panorama from the summit (pages 102 to 123) to carry on your hike. The rest of the book can be a souvenir of a wonderful hike, and you can read the background information at your leisure. If you are backpacking and can take a more leisurely pace, consider carrying the entire book up (it is, after all, only 152 pages). You might find yourself looking at the plants and geologic features along the trail and be pleased to learn more about them. Or, as you eat a snack, you can read a little about the history of Mt. Whitney. Regardless of how you do it, you're sure to fall in love with this iconic peak.

Human History

As a mountaineering destination, a survey point, a scientific laboratory, or simply as the backdrop for western films, Mt. Whitney has long captured people's interest.

EARLY VIEWS OF MT. WHITNEY

The first white men to see Mt. Whitney were probably members of a party led by western explorer Joseph Walker in 1834. They traveled south from the Truckee River, passing through Owens Valley before crossing to the western side of the Sierra Nevada at Walker Pass. However, these men were not surveyors and did not know which of the many peaks along the escarpment was the highest, much less that one peak had the distinction of being taller than the already well-known Cascade volcanoes.

Over the next three decades, as various mining booms occurred, ever more people moved to Owens Valley and the surrounding mountains, but most did not venture deep into the Sierra. It was only on July 2, 1864, when Mt. Whitney was first viewed and surveyed from the west, that it achieved its status as highest in the country. (Whitney relinquished this title in 1959, when Alaska, with its 20,320-foot Denali and 17 other peaks taller than Mt. Whitney, was admitted to the United States.) On that day, William Brewer and Charles Hoffmann, respectively a botanist (and field crew leader) and topographer for the California State Geological Survey, made the first ascent of 13,570-foot Mt. Brewer and saw the layout of the southern High Sierra for the first time, including the location of the tallest peak in the range.

RACE FOR FIRST ASCENT

The race to ascend the high point began two days later. Two other members of the geological survey, Clarence King, a geologist and keen and dare-devilish explorer, and Dick Cotter, an assistant, begged permission to head to the peak. They went through uncharted country: across the Kings-Kern Divide and into the Kern River drainage. Thinking they were heading for the Sierra Nevada's high point, they ascended along what is now called Shepherd Creek, and summited not Whitney but 14,019-foot Mt. Tyndall, the Sierra's eighth-highest peak. From the top, they surveyed the surrounding peaks, noting several that were higher, including Mt.

Whitney. Upon their ascent, King named Mt. Tyndall in honor of a famous British scientist.

Although King and Cotter had to head north to continue their survey after climbing Tyndall, the desire to be the first to summit Mt. Whitney stuck with King. The following day, he received permission to temporarily leave the party and make a second attempt to reach Mt. Whitney. With two cavalrymen and a few horses, he again set out for the Kern River drainage, this time via the Hockett Trail from the San Joaquin Valley. En route, he passed today's Mt. Langley, calling it "Sheeps Peak," and continued to Mt. Whitney. He made it within about 300 feet of the summit, before he had to turn back due to bad weather.

In 1871, King made a third attempt, this time from Owens Valley, via a southern route. In writing about the stormy day when he ascended the "true" summit of Mt. Whitney, King noted what he thought was Mt. Tyndall, some distance to the north. But two years later, a family from Lone Pine climbed this peak, found King's summit note, and informed him that he had actually climbed what is known today as Mt. Langley (his "Sheeps Peak"), some miles south of Mt. Whitney.

It wasn't entirely King's fault, for on his map, the name "Mt. Whitney" was mistakenly attached to Mt. Langley. In 1870, Charles Hoffmann led a survey to the Inyo Mountains, and on maps later created, it was falsely reported that Mt. Langley was Mt. Whitney. Ironically, the error was in part due to King, who made faulty compass measurements from the summit of Mt. Tyndall in 1864. Moreover, Langley and Whitney have similar shapes, and from lower elevations such as the location of Hoffmann's survey team, it is difficult to distinguish which peak is higher. Two meadows on the Kern Plateau to the west of Mt. Langley are a relic of this mapping mistake, as they still hold the name Whitney.

By the 1870s, people from Lone Pine were regularly crossing into the Kern drainage to escape Owens Valley summers. They took the Hockett Trail from the east, crossed the Sierra Crest at Cottonwood Pass, and then traversed the Kern Plateau, before dropping to the Kern River near today's Kern River ranger station, at the southern boundary of Sequoia National Park. In 1873, three men, Charles D. Begole, Albert H. Johnson, and John Lucas, who were camped along the Kern River, decided to leave their fishing camp for a few days and head toward the Sierra Crest. On their trip, they summited

WHITNEY'S "CHANGING" ELEVATION

"Few mountain elevations have been discussed more carefully than that of Mt. Whitney," said meteorologist Alexander McAdie in 1904. The debate continues today.

Over the years, more refined techniques and better estimates of other California elevations have led to more accurate measurements for Mt. Whitney. Estimates have ranged from 14,423 feet to nearly 15,000 feet, and its altitude is currently listed at 14,505 feet.

In 1964, members of the Whitney survey made the first estimates of Mt. Whitney's elevation from the summits of Mt. Brewer and Mt. Tyndall. They used handheld compasses to determine Mt. Whitney's location through triangulation and the vertical angle between their location and Mt. Whitney's summit to determine its elevation. These surveys suggested that the summit stood well above 14,500 feet.

To determine the elevation from the summit itself, the 19th century surveyors carried mercury barometers. Scientists determined the air pressure, temperature, and vapor pressure and compared these results to others simultaneously obtained at a nearby location whose altitude was known. (Accommodating weather was required for acceptable barometer readings, and these early readings were often erroneous.) In this way, Carl Rabe, a member of the third ascent party, made the first summit measurements on September 6, 1873, and estimated Whitney's elevation at 14,898 feet.

This number was quoted in official sources for several decades, but more accurate estimates were soon available, including the Wheeler Survey's 1875 estimate of 14,471 feet, and Samuel Langley's 1881 estimate of 14,522 feet.

A persistent problem with these estimates was the uncertainty of Lone Pine's elevation, one reference point for Mt. Whitney. Langley's 1881 elevation was recalculated to 14,423 feet when a new elevation estimate (based on the railroad grade) for Lone Pine became available.

In 1905, and again in late 1920s, the elevation of Mt. Whitney was determined quite accurately by running leveling lines from Lone Pine to the summit. During the summers of 1925 and 1928, workers with the U.S. Coast and

Geodetic Survey laboriously laid plank upon plank end to end from Lone Pine to the summit to determine horizontal distance. After every few planks, they used a leveling instrument to determine change in elevation, sighting to a 12-foot rod a known distance away. They then added the many incremental increases in elevation. Remarkably, the two surveys done in this way yielded elevations that differed by just 5 feet.

The U.S. Geological Survey (USGS) placed benchmarks on boulders at the summit of Mt. Whitney to indicate these known elevations. Due to the differing heights of each boulder, these benchmarks differ by several feet and do not really represent the height of the mountain. Most of these benchmarks record a height slightly below 14,500 feet.

Today's estimates have become more refined through the use of global positioning system (GPS) devices. Although the handheld devices carried by hikers provide a measurement that is accurate only to about 20 feet, it is possible to get a much more accurate measurement by allowing the GPS units to measure continuously for a longer period of time (e.g., 24 hours).

However, since elevation is a relative term, assigning an elevation to a known vertical position is tricky. Initially, the term implied "elevation above mean sea level," but mean sea level is not the same around the globe. Today, geographic reference systems use an elliptical model of the Earth's surface and measure elevation as a distance above this ellipsoid. The most commonly used reference frame in GPS units is the World Geodetic System 1984 (WGS 1984). The ongoing shifts in reference elevations are responsible for the 1988 change in Mt. Whitney's "official" elevation from 14,497 to 14,505 feet. (Note that the USGS maps still use the National Geodetic Vertical Datum of 1929, and therefore indicate different elevations than those calculated by the more recent National Geodetic Survey.)

Since plate tectonics are probably continuing to push Mt. Whitney slowly skyward, erosive forces are grinding it downward, and geographers are likely to continue refining the shape of their ellipsoid model, the elevation of Whitney is likely to change again.

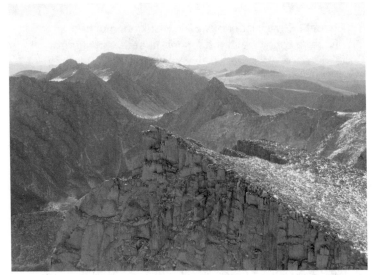

The view south from Mt. Whitney, including from left to right, Mt. Langley, Mt. McAdie, Olancha Peak, and Cirque Peak

first Mt. Langley, and then, on August 18, 1873, they made the first ascent of Mt. Whitney from the southwest. They left the Hockett Trail, traveled north, probably passing the vicinity of Crabtree Meadow, before climbing east toward Mt. Whitney. In subsequent weeks, two more parties successfully climbed Whitney: William Crapo and Abe Leyda in late August, and William Crapo, William L. Hunter, Tom McDonough, and Carl Rabe on September 6, 1873. (The men in the second and third ascent parties attacked the claims made by the three fishermen, but the fishermen's truthful story eventually prevailed.)

Meanwhile, upon hearing that he had ascended the wrong peak in 1871, Clarence King left his survey job on the East Coast and rushed back to California to attempt Whitney again. On September 19, 1873, King finally succeeded, along with partner Frank Knowles, but they had to settle for fourth place.

OTHER EARLY ASCENTS

On October 21, 1873, the naturalist John Muir pioneered a new route from the east that is now known as the Mountaineer's Route. However, for many years, the non-technical route up the western face remained the most popular. Indeed, once the early summiteers showed that it was fairly easy to climb Mt. Whitney from the west, it quickly became a sought-after climb. Parties continued to follow the Hockett Trail across the Sierra Crest and then traveled north via the Kern Plateau, Rock Creek, and Guyot Pass to reach today's Crabtree Meadow. Some parties would reach the summit in a long day from Crabtree Meadow, but most established a higher camp near Guitar Lake. It was via this route that, in the summer of 1878, the first woman, Anna Mills, climbed to the summit.

In 1896, A. W. de la Cour Carroll, a charter member of the Sierra Club from Lone Pine, was the first to describe an ascent via a route similar to today's Mt. Whitney Trail. His party of five men and three women left the vicinity of Outpost Camp early on August 28, 1895, and followed Lone Pine Creek up to Consultation Lake. It appears that from there they climbed toward Whitney Pass (well south of Trail Crest). From there, they descended toward Hitchcock and Guitar lakes, where they spent a night, before climbing the mountain. This circuitous route took them down 2500 feet and then

NAMING OF WHITNEY

Like many great peaks, Mt. Whitney has had a variety of names, and much controversy over its official name. In 1864, the Whitney Survey named the summit Mt. Whitney, to honor Josiah Dwight Whitney, the chief of the California State Geological Survey. However, in 1873, the party that claimed the first ascent—the three fishermen from Lone Pine, Charles Begole, Albert Johnson, and John Lucas— named the peak Fisherman's Peak to memorialize the first ascent of such a significant peak by three "lowly" fishermen.

In fact, any alternative to "Mt. Whitney" was popular among the Lone Pine locals, who were not fond of the mountain's namesake. Trying to pick a less controversial name, Lone Pine's residents temporarily attached the name "Dome of Inyo" to the peak, but then reverted to "Fisherman's Peak." In 1881, a bill was introduced to the California legislature to make "Fisherman's Peak" the official name. It may have been approved, but as an April 1 prank, a legislator changed the proposed name from "Fisherman's Peak" to "Fowler's Peak." As a result, the governor viewed the entire campaign as a farce and vetoed the bill. And so, Mt. Whitney remains the official name.

immediately back up again to avoid a traverse of the pinnacles south of Mt. Whitney's summit. Luckily, on the return, Carroll identified a passable route closer to Trail Crest, shaving time and distance from their descent. Although others took advantage of this route in the following years, most hikers continued to eschew the steep talus chutes up the east face and instead journeyed over Cottonwood Pass. Indeed, the trail from Crabtree Meadow remained incredibly popular: In 1903, a Sierra Club party of 103 ascended via this route.

THE MT. WHITNEY TRAIL

In the early 1900s, Gustave Marsh, a newcomer to Lone Pine, realized that increased Mt. Whitney tourism would benefit the little town, and a more direct trail to the summit might attract more people. Moreover, he envisioned a trail to the summit passable by pack stock. Initially, most townspeople didn't share his enthusiasm, but Marsh nonetheless began fundraising, and before long, Lone Pine citizens pitched in as well, funding much of the work. Letters about the project to Marsh's friend, meteorologist Alexander McAdie, were published in the *Sierra Club Bulletin*, undoubtedly as much to elicit money from its members as to report on progress.

Work on the trail commenced in August of 1903, when a crew of 14 Lone Pine residents built a trail that followed a course similar to the route that A. W. de la Cour Carroll had pioneered nearly a decade earlier. The men toiled to build a route through the field of talus, where moving one boulder often initiated an avalanche of rock that damaged the trail down the slope. When they reached Whitney Pass (just north of Mt. McAdie, a mile southeast of today's Trail Crest), they ran out of funds and work stopped. Two months later, having procured additional funds, they continued working toward the summit. The inhospitable fall weather caused half the workers to abandon the job, and a winter storm in late October forced the others to retreat as well. After an additional 10 days of work the following summer, the trail was completed to the summit on July 18, 1904. The crew celebrated with a large bonfire on top—after all, they now had a trail passable by pack stock, which carried the wood to the summit.

In 1909, plans were made to build a research shelter for the Smithsonian Institution atop Mt. Whitney, requiring that repairs be made to the trail. Marsh received the contract to construct the

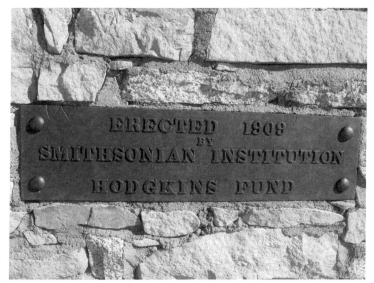

The plaque on the Smithsonian Institution research hut on the summit

summit hut, with the understanding that he would first reestablish the trail where rock slides and avalanches had made the track impassable to stock.

By the early 1920s, however, the trail was again in disrepair due to rockslides, and stock could not reach even the Sierra Crest. Reconstruction began in 1928 as part of an effort to refine the estimated height of Mt. Whitney by leveling from Lone Pine to the summit. Crews from Sequoia National Park worked simultaneously on the Mt. Whitney Trail and on the newly constructed 67-mile High Sierra Trail. By late 1929, stock parties could once again reach the top of Mt. Whitney. In the early 1940s, more work was done on the trail, including the rerouting of the 99 switchbacks to avoid ice fields. Since then, the trail has been maintained, but not much has changed.

What has changed are wilderness ethics. To limit wear on the trail, pack stock were banned in the 1970s, and a camping ban was instituted to protect the fragile lakeshore resources at popular Mirror Lake. Bear canisters are now required, and in 2007, the toilets along the trail were removed and hikers are now required to pack out their solid waste.

ASTRONOMY ATOP MT. WHITNEY

The large number of peaks named for prominent astronomers (see "Namesakes of Whitney-Area Peaks" on page 124) show that astronomy and atmospheric research has had a long history in the Mt. Whitney area. Astronomers require a high-elevation location, with its thinner atmosphere, and the region is ideal, since with its relatively stable weather measurements can be made on most days.

Samuel Langley, the director of the Allegheny Observatory in Pennsylvania, was the first to take advantage of this. In 1881, he made measurements of solar radiation at 11,625 feet, near Guitar Lake, which came to be known as Langley Camp. His assistant James Keeler repeated some of the measurements on the summit of Mt. Whitney. This data allowed Langley to calculate the solar constant, the amount of solar radiation that would reach the Earth's surface in the absence of the atmosphere. Although his calculations were more than twice the correct number, they were the first estimates of this value, and the unit known as the "langley" was designated in 1947 as the international unit of solar radiation.

Alexander McAdie, chief forecaster at the San Francisco office of the U.S. Weather Bureau and vice president of the Sierra Club from 1904 to 1913, became a vocal advocate of Mt. Whitney as an ideal location for a meteorological observatory following a visit to the summit in 1903. In the end, his enthusiasm for mountain weather, his love of the Sierra, and his friendships with nonscientists were more important contributions to the scientific community that were his observations themselves. Without his friendship with Gustave Marsh, the Lone Pine resident who built the original Mt. Whitney Trail, and his many articles in the *Sierra Club Bulletin*, it's unlikely that the summit shelter would have been constructed, and far fewer people would have learned about the results obtained on Mt. Whitney.

Langley's measurements and McAdie's advertisements led W. Wallace Campbell, the longtime director of the Lick Observatory and later the president of the University of California, to consider Mt. Whitney's summit for his research. He decided it was a perfect place from which to determine if the atmosphere on Mars contained water vapor. These measurements had to be made at a location with little water vapor, and a high elevation was necessary because water vapor decreases more rapidly than oxygen with increased elevation. He knew he could only make these observations in late August 1909, when Mars passed close to the Earth. Indeed, it's likely he had been eyeing this location since 1894, the last time Mars's orbit was sufficiently close.

In 1908, together with astronomer Charles Abbot, Campbell made a brief trip to the summit and determined that a cabin was necessary for scientists to remain for longer observation periods. Funds were obtained from the Smithsonian Institute, and Marsh received the contract to upgrade the Mt. Whitney Trail and organize the construction of a research cabin. As with the construction of the trail, Marsh worked efficiently, completing the cabin in less than a month—but still just in time. It was finished on August 27, 1909, and Campbell arrived with his expensive custom instruments the following morning. The measurements he made over the coming days settled the long-running debate, conclusively showing that Mars's atmosphere had, at best, trace amounts of water vapor. Simultaneously, Abbot repeated Langley's solar radiation measurements, obtaining a better estimate of the solar constant. McAdie, the third member of the research party, made meteorological measurements. In 1910, Abbot made additional measurements to refine the solar constant.

The summit hut was built for those few days of observations in August and September 1909, but it saw sporadic use by astronomers and meteorologists over the following decade. In 1910, Marsh ascended the peak to see Halley's comet during a lunar eclipse. In 1913, Abbot's Swedish colleague, A. K. Angström made additional measurements on atmospheric radiation. Since then, the hut has not been used for research and is now just a reminder of the mountain's vibrant history. In 1977, the summit cabin was added to the National Register of Historic Places; it is building #77000119 (see: www.nationalregisterofhistoricplaces.com/CA/Tulare/vacant.html).

Natural History

When you take a walk in nature, you are continuously passing natural history stories captured in the plants, animals, rocks, and sky. These stories have two dimensions. First, each organism or rock you pass is named based on its physical characteristics. However, what you see also holds evidence of past events and ongoing processes. The living organisms along the Mt. Whitney Trail are there because they have adapted to deal with the long, cold, wet winters and the dry summer months. Unlike those in other alpine regions of the world, most of the plant species here evolved from desert-dwelling species. Some traits, like the low stature of alpine plants and the small leaves of plants on dry soil, are visible to every passerby, while other traits are physiological in nature and measured by inquisitive scientists. The rocks, likewise, hold clues to their history. For instance, the chemical composition of the rock informs scientists where the rock originated. This section provides an overview of the natural history along the Mt. Whitney Trail, and I encourage you to observe as you're marching along.

GEOLOGY

The entire Mt. Whitney Trail travels over rock known as the "Whitney granodiorite." Granodiorite is an intrusive igneous rock that originated as molten magma solidified belowground, forming a pluton—an irregular-shaped mass of intrusive rock. Granodiorite is mostly composed of five minerals: quartz, plagioclase (a type of feldspar), potassium feldspar, hornblende, and biotite. The rock's salt-and-pepper-speckled appearance is created by the combination of light-colored quartz and feldspar together with black-colored hornblende and biotite. (Compared to granite, granodiorite has a higher percentage of hornblende and biotite.) Each mineral has a specific chemical composition, shape, hardness, and other characteristics. For instance, the darker-colored minerals have a greater proportion of iron and magnesium than the lighter-colored minerals. In both granodiorite and granite, each mineral's individual crystals are large enough to be visible with the naked eye, indicating the rock cooled relatively slowly.

To understand how the granodiorite formed, we must turn to plate tectonics. The Earth's surface can be divided into at least 15 plates, relatively thin pieces of solid rock (the crust) that float and rotate on the molten material (the mantle) that lies beneath them. As they move, the individual plates may separate, slide past one another, collide, or do any combination of these motions. From about 120 million to 80 million years ago, the Farallon Plate collided with and slid (subducted) beneath the North American Plate. The subducting material was subjected to high temperatures and pressures, causing it and the overlying crust from the North American Plate to melt. Between 88 million and 83 million years ago some of this material solidified into the rock formations that comprise the Whitney Intrusive Suite, a collection of three plutons, including the Whitney granodiorite. These plutons and others comprise the Sierra Nevada batholith (a batholith is a collection of plutons with an exposed surface area greater than 40 square miles).

The crystals comprising the Whitney granodiorite are large compared to the crystals in granites and granodiorites elsewhere in the Sierra. This is because the pluton is nested in the middle of the Whitney Intrusive Suite, where the outer layers of rock provided insulation, which allowed the magma to cool slowly and the individual crystals to grow larger before the magma solidified completely. Especially noteworthy in the Whitney granodiorite are large crystals of potassium feldspar, termed "pegmatites." Rectangular in shape and often measuring 2 inches in each dimension, these crystals protrude from boulders. If you're lucky, you may see a crystal

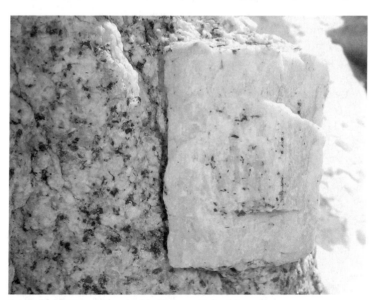

A zoned feldspar crystal embedded in a granite boulder

in which concentric rectangles of small dark crystals are visible. These are small hornblende crystals that were engulfed in the more rapidly growing feldspar. Along the Mt. Whitney Trail, these large crystals are most common on the slope above the John Muir Trail junction.

As you hike up the Mt. Whitney Trail, you are likely to see more geologic features than just the evidence of the plutons. Here are a few of the highlights:

Joints: These natural fractures within the granite formed because the rock contracted as it cooled. The pinnacled profile of the Sierra Crest from Trail Crest to the summit of Mt. Whitney is due to jointing. In addition, the regular, large-scale fractures in the rock between the Hitchcock Lakes and Guitar Lake, on the west side of

HOW WHITNEY GOT ITS HEIGHT

As you climb ever upward, you may wonder how Mt. Whitney got so high. Even today, scientific researchers are debating this complex issue. What they do agree on is that there have been multiple episodes of uplift in the region, each driven by different geologic forces, and each part of the story that created such a tall mountain range.

Emplacement of the plutons caused the initial uplift of a mountain range in this location. This 80-million-year-old "proto-Sierra" was an elevated, rolling landscape and was subsequently worn down by erosion. Nonetheless, evidence of this mountain range remains: The flat summit regions on Mt. Whitney and many surrounding mountains attest to a period when the mountains were less rugged and the valleys less incised.

A second stage of uplift, which initiated the formation of the mountains we see today, began much more recently, probably 10 million years ago. It was around this time that, due to tectonic plate movements, the region east of the Sierra Nevada began to stretch and thin. This motion created a series of faults, or fractures in the rock, that caused valleys to drop down and ridges to rise. This formed the many mountain ranges that exist today in what is appropriately known as the Basin and Range, which extends through Nevada and into Utah. The faults along the eastern

Mt. Whitney, are along joints. On a finer scale, the boulders perched on the summit of Mt. Whitney formed by jointing. Multiple sets of joints caused the rock to fracture into blocks, which eroded to form fairly rounded giant boulders.

Avalanche chutes: These usually form along joints, where the fractured rock is displaced by water that alternately freezes and thaws in the cracks. As a result, the loose rock is carried downslope by gravity, often entrained by snow. These avalanches not only remove rock, but also polish the chutes. In places, giant slides are truncated some distance above today's valley floor, at the boundary between "steep avalanche chute" and "nearly vertical wall." The bottoms of the much older avalanche chutes were cut off by the more recent glaciers, and this transition marks the height to which the valley was

side of the Sierra Nevada are the westernmost extent of this activity, and the Sierra Nevada (or at least its eastern escarpment) can be considered the Basin and Range's westernmost mountain range.

The most recent and most rapid period of uplift began approximately 3.5 million years ago. The main impetus for this uplift appears to have been the breaking off of a large piece from the bottom of the crust. Having dropped some ballast, the remaining, now thinner, crust became more buoyant and rose. The increased buoyancy enhanced the uplift along faults in Owens Valley, increasing the height of the Sierra Crest and therefore Mt. Whitney.

As a result of these events, Mt. Whitney eventually "grew" to nearly 11,000 feet above Owens Valley. But the combined amount of uplift and down-drop on the Sierra Nevada Fault and adjacent Owens Valley Fault are still greater: Bedrock in Owens Valley lies approximately 9000 feet below the Owens Valley floor, indicating Mt. Whitney actually stands 20,000 feet above the rock under the valley floor. The series of faults in Owens Valley are still active— in 1872, Lone Pine was leveled by an earthquake on the Owens Valley Fault that was estimated to be at least 7.5 on the Richter scale. However, most movement on these faults is now horizontal, not vertical, and it is unclear if Mt. Whitney is still growing.

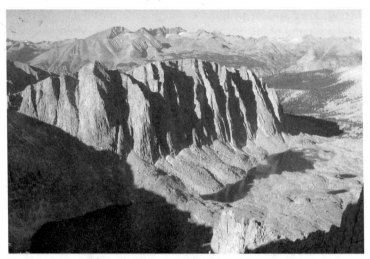

The view southwest from Mt. Whitney, including from left to right, the Hitchcock Lakes, Mt. Hitchcock, and the Kaweah peaks

once filled with ice. Avalanche chutes are obvious on the north face of Mt. Hitchcock, the steep peak to the west of Trail Crest that is seen from Trail Crest to the summit of Mt. Whitney. The boundary between unglaciated and glaciated rock is most obvious if you look north while on the 99 switchbacks: Pinnacle Ridge and the east face of Mt. Whitney were not glaciated, while the basin below was.

Rock glaciers: Like ice glaciers, rock glaciers—rocks that are cemented together by ice—move slowly downslope due to gravity. Rock glaciers are often mistaken for moraines (see next entry), as both appear to be poorly sorted collections of boulders. However, rock glaciers are characterized by a notable steep front and often a flattish, rippled top. Along the Mt. Whitney Trail, there are several large rock glaciers in the basin east of Mt. Whitney, including one just to the northwest of Trail Camp. Their U shapes are readily visible as you approach the cables on the 99 switchbacks.

Moraines: These ridges formed by the accumulation of rocks and other debris that was carried downslope by a glacier. Lateral moraines form along the sides of the valley, while a terminal moraine marks the farthest down-valley extent of the glacier. Along the Mt. Whitney Trail, most moraines have been overrun by rock glaciers.

Glacial polish: These smooth, shiny surfaces are created when the sediment at the bottom of a glacier is scraped across rock outcrops, evening and smoothing them, and leaving a shiny surface. However, coarse rocks dragged along by the glacier may leave grooves and striations. Hunt for sections of glacial polish as you walk along the ridge a little below Trailside Meadow.

JOSIAH DWIGHT WHITNEY

As the supervisor of the California State Geological Surveys (the "Whitney Surveys") between 1860 and 1864, Josiah Dwight Whitney played an important role in the scientific history of the Sierra Nevada. Appointed California state geologist in 1860, he assembled an impressive team of scientists from all disciplines—topography, botany, and geology—to explore and survey the state.

When the surveyors mapped the Sierra during the summers of 1863 and 1864, they were the first nonnatives to visit the southern High Sierra. From the summit of Mt. Brewer, they were also the first white men to see the state's highest peak from the west, and they named it after their boss.

The members of the Whitney Surveys studied all aspects of California natural history, not just the locations of mineral resources. Unfortunately, California state legislators cared most about finding the location of gold and abolished the survey in 1865 when their interests weren't realized. Whitney retained the title of state geologist until 1874, but he returned to the East Coast in 1865 for a professorship at Harvard University.

Today, Whitney is often remembered only for his erroneous belief that Yosemite Valley was not glaciated but created when the valley floor "down-dropped." This led to a lifelong dispute with famous naturalist John Muir, who argued that glaciation was the main mechanism responsible for shaping the Sierra Nevada's landscapes. As the person with greater political power, Whitney forcefully told others that Muir was ignorant and incorrect, stalling the acceptance of Muir's observations, which were later accepted as *mostly* accurate. Whitney was, however, a well-respected, moral scientist—just one who was unwilling to admit a key mistake.

VEGETATION

Climbing up more than 6000 feet takes you through four vegetation zones, each of which can be further divided based on the slope's aspect and steepness. Depending on temperature, moisture availability, and other factors, these zones either begin and end abruptly or grade into one another.

Montane Zone: Whitney Portal lies in the Montane Zone, which, in the southern Sierra, extends from about 7500 feet to just above 9000 feet. Along the Mt. Whitney Trail, white firs and Jeffrey pines dominate the forested sections of this zone. However, due to the steep aspect and dry soils at this elevation range along the trail, you will mostly be walking through the montane chaparral community. Drought-resistant evergreen shrubs such as mountain mahogany and bush chinquapin are common members of the community.

Subalpine Zone: The Subalpine Zone is loosely defined as a region where tree cover thins, although forest cover can still exist—from around 9500 to 11,000 feet in elevation in the Whitney region. The understory is usually sparse and the soils poor. In the southern Sierra, this zone is dominated by lodgepole pine, foxtail pine, and whitebark pine, the latter of which is rare along the Mt. Whitney Trail. On flatter slopes, such as near Lone Pine Lake, a dense monostand of lodgepole pine is common, while tree cover lessens and foxtail pines become more common in steeper areas. The latter is an important member of the subalpine community only in the southern Sierra. The Subalpine Zone ends where trees can no longer establish. Along this trail, you will find the last trees about half a mile above Mirror Lake.

Alpine Zone: The Alpine Zone begins above timberline, usually around 11,000 feet in the southern Sierra, and includes only shrubs, herbs, and grasses. In regions with sufficient water, you may encounter meadows, a plant community found along the Mt. Whitney Trail only at Trailside Meadow and near Trail Camp. Meadows have a dense cover of grass interspersed with a collection of wildflowers. Elsewhere, ground cover is sparser. In the Alpine Zone, species composition can be quite varied, depending on small differences in location, as each species has individual requirements for establishment and growth. Many species grow alongside boulders, with their roots seeking the moister soil beneath the rock. Cushion plants are common in sandy flats between rocks, as growing close to the ground alleviates wind chill and the temperatures can be many degrees warmer. As the elevation increases and the growing conditions deteriorate, the species diversity declines.

Barren Rock: At the highest elevations, no plants can survive. On north-facing slopes, the growing season may be too short, for winter snows may remain on the ground long into summer. On exposed, west-facing slopes, the winter temperatures may be too extreme, as winter winds often strip such slopes of all insulating snow cover. Along the last mile to the summit of Mt. Whitney, even the sky pilot and alpine gold disappear, as a combination of winter temperatures, winter winds, and growing season length make the environment too stressful.

Since the Mt. Whitney Trail traverses so many vegetation zones, there is a rich diversity of more than 150 plant species growing alongside the trail. The following is a small subset of species that grow along the trail. They were selected to represent the species you are most likely to notice—some are common along the trail for considerable distances, while others appear only a few places but are abundant and hard to miss. There is a bias toward the higher-elevation species, for it is at these elevations that you will be going most slowly and likely staring at the ground.

For each species, I have provided the common name and scientific name (in parentheses). The species are listed in the approximate order they appear along the Mt. Whitney Trail. This is followed by a brief description to aid in identifying the species.

When at home, check out the following website, which is a wonderful resource with color photos of many of California's plants: http://calphotos.berkeley.edu/flora.

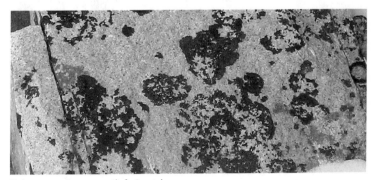

Lichens growing on north-facing talus

HERBS AND SHRUBS

Mountain mahogany *(Cercocarpus ledifolius)*: This large shrub dots the slopes adjacent to the trail from the start up to approximately 9200 feet. It becomes less common about halfway between the North Fork of Lone Pine Creek crossing and the Lone Pine Lake junction. It has small, oval-shaped, leathery leaves, but it is most easily distinguished beginning midseason when it is covered with distinctive seeds: Each seed bears a 1-inch, curled tail that is densely covered in branched hairs. These hairs catch the light, giving the entire plant a wonderful glow.

Fernbush *(Chamaebatiaria millefolium)*: A common large shrub that grows between Whitney Portal and the top of the dry slopes below the Lone Pine Lake junction, this species is named for its much-dissected leaves that resemble fern fronds. The dark green foliage has a strong odor and is covered with glands and hairs. Its five white petals ring a dense cluster of yellow stamens, the pollen-producing male reproductive parts.

Sierra angelica *(Angelica lineariloba)*: A member of the carrot family, Sierra angelica is common on the slope leading to the Lone Pine Lake junction. Usually 3 to 4 feet tall, it bares many small, white flowers in a large, spherical head. As indicated by its scientific name, its leaves are dissected into long, linear lobes.

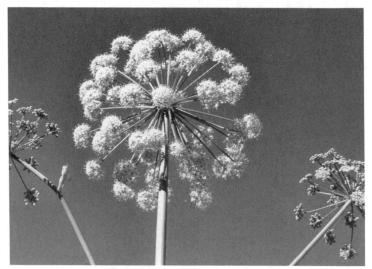

Sierra angelica *(Angelica lineariloba)*

Scarlet penstemon *(Penstemon rostriflorus)*: There are many spe-cies of penstemon in the Sierra Nevada, inhabiting environments from wet meadows to high sandy plateaus. The flowers come in all shades of reds, purples, and blues, and are always identifiable by their long, tubular flowers. In the Sierra Nevada, the scarlet penste-mon (or Bridge's penstemon) is the species with the most vibrant red flowers attached to a single long stalk. It is present on many dry, sandy slopes up to 10,500 feet. The Mt. Whitney Trail is no excep-tion, and although this species is present until you reach Mirror Lake, it is especially common below the Lone Pine Lake junction.

Rothrock's beardtongue *(Keckiella rothrockii)*: A relative of the penstemons, this light pink, flowered herb is common from Whitney Portal until a short distance before the South Fork of Lone Pine Creek crossing. The flowers are smaller and wider than those of scarlet penstemon, but they are likewise tubular.

Inyo meadow lupine *(Lupinus pratensis)*: This tall lupine occurs in the wet area just downstream of the first crossing of Lone Pine Creek. A member of the pea family, it has mostly purple flowers on elongate flowering stalks. Its 5 to 10 leaflets are each 1 to 3 inches long and fuse to a single point—making it palmate, like your hand. The peapod-like fruits are hairy to woolly.

Mouse-tail ivesia *(Ivesia santolinoides)*: Along the Mt. Whitney Trail, you will see this species only once, but you can't miss the large cluster of these dainty white flowers near the Mt. Whitney Zone sign (just beyond the Lone Pine Lake junction). The leaves of this species certainly resemble mouse tails, with 2- to 4-inch stalks of densely clustered, very tiny, and hairy leaflets. Each flower sits atop a loosely branched, long stalk, and each of the five petals resembles a miniature rose petal—indeed, this species is a member of the rose family.

Wavy-leaved paintbrush *(Castilleja applegatei)*: A common spe-cies on dry slopes throughout the Sierra Nevada from 4000 to 11,000 feet, this paintbrush grows along the Mt. Whitney Trail up to around Mirror Lake. It is especially common on the switchbacks just after you enter the Mt. Whitney Zone and again on the switch-backs above Outpost Camp. It has heads of red-orange tubular flowers, but if you look closely, you'll see that much of the color is not from the flower but from the tips of the lobed leaves below each flower. This species can always be distinguished from other paintbrushes by its wavy-margined leaves.

Bush chinquapin *(Chrysolepis sempervirens)***:** This shrub, a relative of oaks, grows from Whitney Portal to Mirror Lake. The backside of the leathery leaves is a beautiful golden color, and the fruit is a spiny sphere. It is hard to miss on the switchbacks between Outpost Camp and Mirror Lake.

Mountaineer's shooting star *(Dodecatheon redolens)***:** A common species in wet meadows throughout the Subalpine and Alpine zones of the Sierra Nevada, the mountaineer's shooting star finds few appropriate habitats along the Mt. Whitney Trail. You are most likely to notice it in Trailside Meadow, where it is the dominant herb. Its stalks are approximately a foot tall, and its narrow leaves, which attach to the base of the plant, are nearly that long. Its eponymous flowers have five bent-back lavender petals, the trail of the shooting star. The yellow petal bases are fused together, and the stigma and bulky stamens, the female and male reproductive structures, form the tip of the shooting star.

Cliffbush *(Jamesia americana)***:** Appropriately named cliffbush is a light pink, flowered shrub that often grows in cracks in the cliffs. It has small leaves with serrate tips, and its spreading branches often hug slabs of rock, reminiscent of fruit trees grown as an espalier. Along the Mt. Whitney Trail, cliffbush is common between 11,000 and 12,000 feet, mostly along the north-facing sides of outcrops.

Sierra primrose *(Primula suffrutescens)***:** This is one of the Sierra's most cheerful flowers, with five bright magenta petals that fuse into a yellow ring. This low-growing shrub emerges at the edge of boulders along the Mt. Whitney Trail, mostly between Trailside Meadow and Trail Camp, although a few individuals also grow on the switchbacks above the Mt. Whitney Zone sign. The small, slightly fan-shaped leaves have a serrate outer edge.

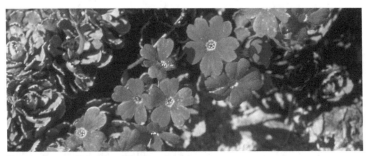

Sierra primrose *(Primula suffrutescens)*

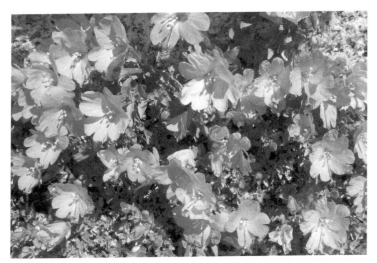

Rockfringe *(Epilobium obcordatum)*

Rockfringe *(Epilobium obcordatum)*: Rockfringe joins the Sierra primrose beneath boulders between Trailside Meadow and Trail Camp. It, too, has bright magenta flowers, but its flowers have four large, very thin petals. A late-blooming species with quite small leaves, it just emerges when most other species are already blooming, and its abundant flowers appear in late summer, as the others fade.

Wax currant *(Ribes cereum)*: This shrub, also called squaw currant, is present along the trail from about 11,000 to 12,500 feet, disappearing as you approach the section of the switchbacks with the handrail. Like all currants, its leaves resemble maple leaves, but with more rounded lobes. By midsummer, the plant bears small, red berries that are edible but not particularly tasty. Unlike most other currants at lower elevations, this species does not have thorns.

Mountain monkeyflower *(Mimulus tilingii)*: Of the approximately 40 species of monkeyflowers in the Sierra Nevada, this is one of the three species you will encounter frequently at high elevations. Along the Mt. Whitney Trail, it is common between Trailside Meadow and Trail Camp. Its yellow flowers are tubular, with two petals attached above and three petals arranged below the tube's red-spotted mouth. (The central petal on the bottom is lobed, giving the appearance of two petals.) As with many monkeyflowers, this species grows near trickles of water, both alongside streams and under moist overhangs.

Oval-leaved buckwheat (Eriogonum ovalifolium): This cushion plant becomes common just beyond Trail Camp, growing in sandy patches between boulders. The leaves are densely covered in fine hairs, giving the leaf blades a frosted appearance. Spherical heads of small white flowers are born on 2- to 4-inch stalks. The heads turn pink or reddish by late season, as the flowers go to seed.

Cut-leaf daisy (Erigeron compositus): This small daisy is common throughout the switchbacks. It is best identified by its three-lobed leaves (half inch to an inch in size), because the flowers come in two different forms: Some are characteristic little daisies, with bright yellow centers surrounded by purple rays, but many individuals lack the rays.

Gray chickensage (Sphaeromeria cana): Also known as "tansy," this relative of the sagebrush grows along the bottom half of the switchbacks (between 12,000 and 13,000 feet), though you may spot a few straggling individuals west of Trail Crest. This small shrub grows in sandy patches between boulders on talus fields. It has a disc of minute, cream-colored flowers, which, from a distance, appears as a single, small head with no rays, reminiscent of a button.

Granite draba (Draba lemmonii): This member of the mustard family, common along the 99 switchbacks, is a cushion plant, and hugs rocks, especially near small trickles of water. The tiny oval-shaped leaves are distinguished by their long, hairy edges. In early season, the often large mats are covered with small, yellow, four-petal flowers.

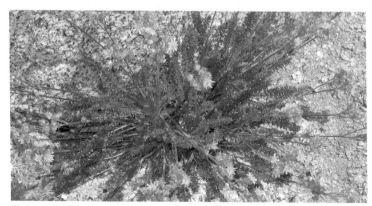

Club-moss ivesia (Ivesia lycopodioides)

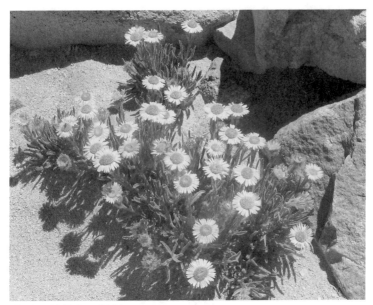

Alpine gold *(Hulsea algida)*

Club-moss ivesia *(Ivesia lycopodioides)*: Like the lower-elevation mouse-tail ivesia, this species has stalks of closely clustered miniature leaflets. However, the leaves of the club-moss ivesia are not hairy and are therefore a brighter green. Its five-petal, yellow flowers are borne at the end of approximately 4-inch stalks, which emerge from a basal cluster of leaves. Along the Mt. Whitney Trail, club-moss ivesia grows mostly at the highest elevations and is most commonly seen toward the top of the switchbacks and near the junction with the John Muir Trail. At these high elevations, it often emerges from cracks in slabs, while at lower elevations it is common in wet meadows.

Alpine gold *(Hulsea algida)*: A type of daisy, alpine gold becomes common around 12,500 feet and grows nearly to the summit of Mt. Whitney. While most of the species along the switchbacks are small (and bear small flowers), alpine gold has large yellow flowers on 6- to 8-inch stalks. Its rather thick leaves are long, narrow, and gland-dotted, with slightly wavy margins. Despite its strong odor, this species is a favorite food of bighorn sheep and pikas. Along the final miles to the summit, you may encounter small piles of clipped alpine gold leaves. These "hay piles" are left by pikas who make them to dry the leaves for winter storage.

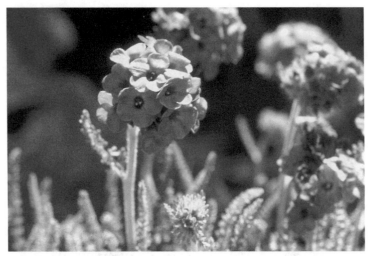

Sky pilot *(Polemonium eximium)*

Sky pilot *(Polemonium eximium)*: Along the Mt. Whitney Trail, alpine gold shares the highest habitats with sky pilot. The showiest of High Sierra species, the sky pilot boasts a 2- to 3-inch diameter, spherical head of vibrant purple flowers. The leaves are deeply dissected, have a pungent odor, and are covered with small glands. This species grows among the cliffs on some of the Sierra's highest peaks and is another favorite food of bighorn sheep and pikas.

TREES

White fir *(Abies concolor)*: Growing from Whitney Portal up to around 9000 feet, the white fir, like all firs, is easily distinguished from pine trees: Its needles attach singly to the branches, instead of being bundled into clusters called fascicles. The needles are well over an inch in length, and the bark of the older trees is light in color. Don't expect to find any fir cones lying on the ground, as the squirrels shred them before they fall.

Jeffrey pine *(Pinus jeffreyi)*: The Jeffrey pines are the towering trees at Whitney Portal that grace the slope all the way up to about 9000 feet. Its long needles are clustered in groups of three, and its large, oval cones are "gentle"—meaning that the tips of the cone's scales are turned inward. Jeffrey pines rarely form a continuous forest cover; instead, they occur singly or in small groups, mostly on dry slopes.

Lodgepole pine *(Pinus contorta)*: The lodgepole pine is the most common tree in the subalpine Sierra Nevada, forming near monocultures on many flats and on some slopes between 9000 and 11,000 feet. Along the Mt. Whitney Trail, the lodgepole pine is most common for the half mile below the Lone Pine Lake junction, although it occurs occasionally to above Mirror Lake. It is distinguished by needles that are borne in clusters of two; fine, scaly bark; and approximately 1.5-inch pinecones that are usually abundant at the base of trees.

Foxtail pine *(Pinus balfouriana)*: The foxtail pine is a southern Sierra species, and some of the largest stands occur on the west side of Mt. Whitney. Along the Mt. Whitney Trail, the beautiful trees are especially prominent at Outpost Camp, with some individuals that appear at elevations of about 11,000 feet, above Mirror Lake. These pines are distinguished by their long, dangling branches that often have needles only near the tip. The needles encircle the stem like a bottlebrush, much like their relatives, the bristlecone pines. Needles are in clusters of five, and cones are about 3 inches long.

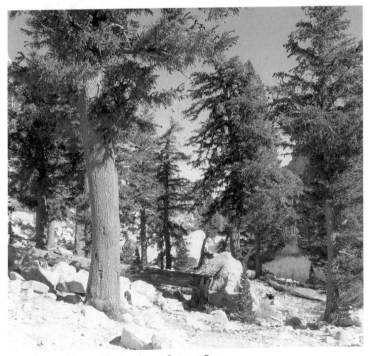

Foxtail pines *(Pinus balfouriana)* near Outpost Camp

ANIMALS

Although more than a dozen mammals and at least 50 bird species inhabit the Mt. Whitney region, as you traverse the landscape, it appears nearly devoid of wildlife. Most mammals eschew human corridors, and many are nocturnal. Although many bird species are present, they are often seen only at dawn and dusk and even then only identified with the aid of binoculars. Nonetheless, it's difficult to ascend Mt. Whitney without seeing a few common alpine (and subalpine) animals and birds. They may include any of the following:

Yellow-bellied marmots: The largest mammal commonly seen, the marmot is technically a large, heavy-set ground squirrel, approximately 2 feet in length (including its bushy tail). In the mid-elevations of the Alpine Zone, marmots are commonly seen lazing atop boulders, flattening their fat bellies into a thick pancake. They are very common (and aggressive) at Trail Camp.

Golden-mantled ground squirrels: About a foot in length, approximately a third of which is tail, this squirrel, unlike the chipmunk, does not have stripes on its head: The distinct white and black stripes extend only to its neck. Their range doesn't extend beyond 10,000 feet, so you will see them only along the lower reaches of the Mt. Whitney Trail.

Alpine chipmunks: These tiny, skinny critters are just 6 to 7 inches in length and are easily identified by their small size and face stripes. The highest-elevation chipmunk, they range above 10,000 feet.

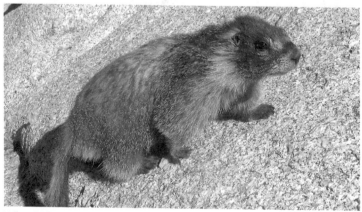

Yellow-bellied marmot

Pikas: These softball-sized balls of fluff have adorable Mickey Mouse ears. Relatives of rabbits, when startled, they emit a "peep-peep"—often the first evidence of their presence, as they quickly scamper into a talus pile. Unlike the rodents, pikas do not hibernate during the winter. Instead, they subsist beneath the talus on plants they have collected during the summer. If you see a pile of cut plant stems sitting on a rock, this is a pika's hay pile being dried for winter.

Bighorn sheep: Infrequently seen along the Mt. Whitney Trail, the bighorn sheep near Mt. Whitney are from the Mt. Langley population, to the south, and wander as far north as Arc Pass, overlooking Consultation Lake. However, they rarely stray any closer to the trail. To the north, members of the Mt. Williamson population have been seen a little south of Vacation Pass, many miles north of the Mt. Whitney Trail.

Grey-crowned rosy finches: Usually observed in small flocks, these finches fly around the alpine landscape in pursuit of insects carried to high elevations by wind currents. When mayfly larvae are hatching into adults, the finches congregate around lakes, gorging themselves. Usually shy, individuals at Trail Camp are remarkably tame as they hop around in search of food.

Common ravens: Usually flying alone or in small groups to the top of Mt. Whitney, these jet black ravens with stout beaks will approach your food at Trail Camp.

Dark-eyed juncos: These sparrows, ubiquitous up to and a bit above the treeline, dart in and out of vegetation and are easily distinguished by their blackish heads contrasting against a brownish-grayish body.

SOUTHERN SIERRA WEATHER

The southern Sierra Nevada, which includes Mt. Whitney, lies between California's Central Valley and Nevada's Great Basin, where it is primarily influenced by weather from the Pacific Ocean. As a result, it experiences a Mediterranean climate with relatively mild, wet winters, and warm, dry summers. From November to March, Pacific storms bring snow and cold, stormy weather, with temperatures lower than −20°F in the regions above 10,000 feet. By April, the ferocity of storms declines, and May heralds the return of warm daytime temperatures. However, nights are still chilly, and a large snow pack usually limits access to the backcountry to well-outfitted mountaineers.

In summer, days are often cloudless and temperatures are warm. During July and August, high temperatures are consistently in the 60s at 11,000 feet, with the warmest days creeping toward the mid-70s. The abundant sunshine can make the temperatures feel even warmer. Summer moisture is rare, with rainfall at Crabtree Meadow (a few miles west of Mt. Whitney) usually totaling just a few inches between mid-June and mid-September.

The summer moisture the Sierra does receive comes up from the south, in remnants of tropical storms originating in the Gulf of California, the southeast Pacific, and even the Gulf of Mexico. Much of the time, this translates into a slow buildup of puffy cumulus clouds, which arrive a bit earlier each afternoon and look a bit more menacing. After a few days, afternoon thunderstorms arrive for a day or two, and then the system disappears again. At times, former tropical cyclones may be entrained in southerly airflow, bringing a larger pulse of moisture to the eastern Sierra. This can result in either a rapid buildup of clouds and/or rain for many hours on end—sometimes even breaking the cardinal rule that "it never rains at night in the Sierra." Any thunderstorm could bring hail to the higher elevations of the Mt. Whitney Trail. More important, the lightning that accompanies these storms presents a serious risk to hikers on the exposed upper section of the Mt. Whitney Trail (see more about precautions during lightning storms on page 45).

And of course, when it comes to weather, there is no such thing as normal, only averages, as the astronomer Charles Abbot once noted following a very wet stormy period in August 1909: "One thing was sure, and that was that seasons differ, and while as a rule that location is dry during summer and fall, there are occasional seasons when this is not the case and the 'land of little rain' has to be taken with a grain of salt."

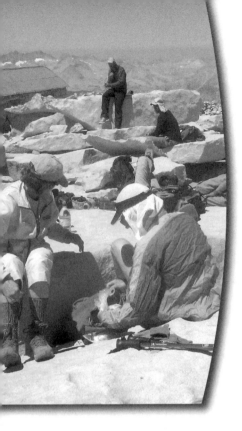

2

Precautions and Considerations

While a hike up the Mt. Whitney Trail is generally considered a fairly safe endeavor, there are some things you should take into account before departing from Whitney Portal. All of the major concerns are outlined in this chapter. Indeed, all of the items listed (even bears, though rarely) do injure people on this trail each year. Some of the concerns described here are serious medical issues that can result in an emergency situation (e.g. hypothermia and altitude sickness), while others are mostly nuisances (e.g. blisters). However, since all can keep you from reaching the summit, you'll want to minimize their impact on your trip and learn to recognize early on when discomfort can morph into a dangerous condition.

Perhaps it's because of my background in science, but when I am in the mountains, I like to remind myself of the term "homeostasis." It is defined as the maintenance of a stable internal environment in the body, despite changes in the external environment. As you hike up Mt. Whitney, the external environment is constantly shifting: Oxygen availability and temperature decrease with altitude, but your cells need constant amounts of oxygen and your internal

Above: Enjoying a hard-earned lunch on the summit of Mt. Whitney   **33**

ACCIDENTS AND INJURIES IN THE SIERRA

If you need one last push to read this section, visit the websites described below. They provide you with real-life stories of injury and death in the Sierra Nevada and generally strike home the reality of dangers in ways describing the medical conditions cannot. The Inyo Country Search and Rescue Team website provides details of many accidents and rescues that have occurred on Mt. Whitney (and other Sierra peaks) since approximately 2003 (see www.inyosar.org, and look under "missions"). In addition, the "What can go wrong on Mt. Whitney" topic on the Whitney Portal Store website (www.whitneyportalstore.com; thread number 39077) is a great source of information.

temperature must be maintained at a constant level. In addition, your blood sugar must be maintained, and the concentration of sodium ions, potassium ions, and many other ions must also be maintained at a constant level. Although the body does a very good job fine-tuning internal conditions, you have to supply it with the essential materials: oxygen, food, and water.

It is also important that you have the knowledge, experience, and gear to appropriately respond to changes in your external environment. This section covers the essential considerations you need to make to avoid physiological problems like altitude sickness, hypothermia, dehydration, electrolyte depletion, as well as other potential hazards like lightning, injuries, blisters, and bears.

Altitude Sickness

The International Society for Mountain Medicine, a group that encourages research on and shares information about mountain medicine, advises its members to abide by its first golden rule of visiting alpine environments: "If you feel unwell at altitude, it is altitude illness until proven otherwise." Altitude sickness is the hazard most likely to affect you on your hike up Mt. Whitney. According to one study conducted during July and August 2006, more than half of the people attempting to summit Mt. Whitney via the Mt. Whitney Trail suffered from the form of altitude sickness known as

Acute Mountain Sickness (AMS), a collection of symptoms, including a headache, that occur when a person rapidly ascends to high altitude.

Many people on the Mt. Whitney Trail plan a rapid ascent (and descent), thinking they don't need to worry about the more severe forms of altitude sickness, High Altitude Cerebral Edema (HACE) and High Altitude Pulmonary Edema (HAPE), because these *usually* take more than 12 hours to develop. Just keep the "usually" in mind; there are cases of HACE and HAPE along the Mt. Whitney Trail, and they often require emergency evacuations. Even relatively mild AMS can impair your judgment, and there is no way to quantify how many accidents are due to poor decisions people made because of AMS.

What follows is a description of how the body responds to decreased oxygen availability and a summary of the symptoms of AMS, HACE, and HAPE. This information is an overview only; if you wish to learn more, I strongly recommend Charles Houston's *Going Higher* (Mountaineers Books, 2005) and the website of the International Society for Mountain Medicine: www.ismmed.org/np_altitude_tutorial.htm.

CAUSES OF ALTITUDE SICKNESS

The root cause of altitude sickness is hypoxia, the insufficient supply of oxygen to the body's tissues. The Earth's atmosphere becomes thinner at higher elevations because, with increasing altitude, there is less weight, and therefore less pressure, exerted by the atmosphere above. As a result, the air at high elevation is lower density than the air at sea level, and thus gasses in the atmosphere, including oxygen, are more spread out. At the summit of Mt. Whitney, there is 58 percent as much oxygen in a given volume as there is at sea level.

Hemoglobin is the protein in red blood cells that carries oxygen to all of the body's cells. As the partial pressure of oxygen in the air you breathe decreases, the amount of oxygen hemoglobin carries to your cells decreases, hence the hypoxia.

In response to the low barometric pressure and low oxygen pressure, the body secretes stress hormones, which affect different parts of the body differently. In the brain, stress hormones cause increased blood flow and hence increased blood supply (and blood pressure) to the capillaries, the smallest blood vessels, in the brain. The increased blood pressure causes the capillaries to leak, which leads to swelling (edema) of the brain tissue. HACE occurs when this swelling is particularly severe. In the lungs, the elevated stress hormone activity causes constriction of the pulmonary vessels, thus increasing resistance to blood flow. In some cases, this leads to increased fluid leakage from the capillaries into the tissues and air spaces (alveoli) in the lungs, reducing the area across which gas exchange can occur and causing HAPE. Also contributing to the body's responses to hypoxia are hormones secreted from the kidney that cause sodium (salt) retention, which in turn causes fluid retention and swollen hands and feet.

Age, genetic factors, level of exertion, and the elevation at which you live appear to be the best predictors of susceptibility to altitude sickness. Anecdotal evidence suggests that teenagers and young adults are more susceptible to altitude sickness than young children or older adults. However, altitude sickness is fickle, affecting the same person differently on different occasions. Even very fit people get altitude sickness. All of which indicates physicians still don't know what makes a person prone to altitude sickness. One study showed that people with more space between their brains and skulls are less susceptible to altitude sickness, because their brain can swell a little without pushing against their skull.

SYMPTOMS OF ALTITUDE SICKNESS

Acute Mountain Sickness (AMS) is actually a collection of symptoms on a continuum that, at its more severe end, includes High Altitude Cerebral Edema (HACE). If you are at high elevation, you by definition have AMS if you have a headache together with one or more of the following symptoms:

- loss of appetite, nausea, or vomiting
- fatigue or weakness
- dizziness or light-headedness
- difficulty sleeping

Other symptoms that may occur when you have AMS include apathy, paleness or sick appearance, shortness of breath, low urine output, and edema of the ankles.

HOW THE BODY ACCLIMATES TO HYPOXIA

The body uses many interlinked processes to compensate for hypoxia, some immediate and some longer term. These allow most individuals to successfully acclimatize to elevations of about 17,000 feet over the course of a month. On a long weekend climb of Mt. Whitney, your body will just be starting to adjust, which is why it is important to begin acclimatizing in advance. Three processes important to acclimation are:

Hyperventilation: At higher elevations, there are fewer oxygen molecules in each breath. This leads to an increased rate of breathing, known as the "hypoxic ventilatory response." This continues for many weeks at altitude and is very important for maintaining higher blood oxygen levels.

Increased blood alkalinity and increased output of bicarbonate in urine: Breathing faster causes the blood to offload more carbon dioxide to the capillaries in the lungs, increasing blood alkalinity (higher pH). However, higher blood pH leads to a negative feedback response: a decreased rate of breathing countering the hypoxic ventilatory response. Since the body needs to maintain the high breathing rate to take in more oxygen, it must counter the higher blood pH. It does this by excreting bicarbonate, an alkaline compound, via the kidneys, shifting blood alkalinity back toward normal. This relatively slow response continues for several days and is probably the main form of acclimation on a trip that lasts between a few days to a week.

The prescription drug acetalzolamide speeds up this process (and allows it to begin at low elevations) by increasing bicarbonate excretion and by increasing blood carbon dioxide levels, thus causing increased ventilation and increased intake of oxygen. It is also a diuretic and enhances sodium excretion, helping to decrease peripheral swelling.

Increased red blood cell count: Although this response begins immediately, it takes your body many weeks to increase its red blood cell count sufficiently to offset the decrease in oxygen pressure.

'E, a severe form of AMS, is characterized by more acute
\a in the brain. In addition to more extreme symptoms of
AMS, individuals with HACE have mental confusion and a loss
of coordination. If a member of your party appears to be develop-
ing these symptoms (e.g. cannot walk in a straight line), he or she
must descend immediately. HACE can lead to death within hours
to days.

HAPE symptoms include a cough, decreased performance, chest
congestion, and shortness of breath while at rest. The often men-
tioned symptoms of severe respiratory distress, coughing of blood,
and gurgling sounds in the chest occur later in the progression of
the condition. As with HACE, an individual with these symptoms
must descend rapidly. The greatest number of altitude sickness
fatalities are due to HAPE. HAPE is more common in men than in
women and can appear in people well acclimatized to high elevations who have descended to low elevations for just a few days and
then reascend.

PREVENTING ALTITUDE SICKNESS

There are many actions you can take to reduce the likelihood of
AMS symptoms:

- **Stay well-hydrated.**
- **Eat enough food.**
- **Ascend slowly.** Although it is rarely followed by hikers on
  the Mt. Whitney Trail, the often-stated rule for diminishing
  risk of AMS is that, above 10,000 feet, you should ascend no
  more than 1000 feet per night. This suggests that overnight
  hikers should spend one night at Outpost Camp, and then
  a second night at Trail Camp before continuing to the summit. Most people will choose not to adopt this plan for Mt.
  Whitney, since it takes an extra day to reach the summit.
  However, if you have a history of AMS, an ascent spread over
  more days might help.
- **Get a good night's sleep before your hike.** Don't drive up
  after work, arrive in Lone Pine at 1 AM, and begin hiking a
  few hours later.
- **Take the time to acclimatize.** On page 56, there are suggestions of nearby dayhikes that take you to elevations of 10,000
  and 12,000 feet. Going high during the day and then sleeping at lower elevations helps your body acclimatize faster

and generally makes you feel better, because at night you'll be able to sleep and eat well. Sleeping low does not mean you have to retreat to Lone Pine for the night. You should plan to sleep at Whitney Portal (elevation 8330 feet) before your hike if you plan on camping. Most people sleep well at Whitney Portal, which allows the body to continue acclimatizing for their excursion up the Mt. Whitney Trail.

- **If you do experience altitude sickness on your hike,** follow the International Society for Mountain Medicine's second golden rule: "Never ascend with symptoms of AMS." Since more than a third of people climbing Mt. Whitney experience AMS symptoms before reaching the summit, many people clearly ignore this advice each year. Yet very few develop symptoms indicative of HAPE or HACE, probably due to the short period of time hikers are at the highest elevations. If you choose to continue upward in spite of AMS symptoms, be aware of the risks, monitor yourself (and have your hiking partners monitor you), and descend immediately if your symptoms worsen.

MEDICAL TREATMENTS FOR ALTITUDE SICKNESS

Although it's by no means necessary if you prepare and acclimate properly, many people climbing Mt. Whitney elect to take medication—mostly aspirin/ibuprofen, and occasionally prescription drugs—in hopes of decreasing their susceptibility to altitude sickness. Some of these medications are described below. Note: I do not recommend taking medications to prevent altitude sickness. If you choose to pursue any drugs, prescription or otherwise, please do so under the care of a medical doctor, and be sure to research the contraindications and side effects of any medication you plan to take.

Aspirin and ibuprofen: Both of these anti-inflammatory drugs help relieve headaches, although many people prefer ibuprofen because it is effective in smaller doses. Taking an anti-inflammatory drug prophylactically may prevent you from feeling lousy due to a headache. If you feel better, you also tend to eat and drink more, which may further minimize altitude sickness.

Acetazolamide: This prescription medication (the main brand name is Diamox) gives your body a head start acclimatizing by acidifying your blood. Common side effects include more frequent urination and a tingling sensation in your toes and fingers. People who are sensitive to sunlight or sulfa drugs may have additional side effects and should consult a doctor about their allergies and sensitivities.

Dexamethasone: This prescription drug is a corticosteroid thought to stabilize edema in blood vessels. It may therefore decrease brain swelling and is used to treat severe symptoms of AMS and HACE, but not HAPE. Dexamethasone is usually carried on high-altitude expeditions. Some doctors also prescribe it as a preventative medicine against altitude sickness. Side effects can include an upset stomach, high blood sugar, and mood changes.

Hypothermia

Hypothermia is a potentially lethal condition that results from an abnormally low body temperature. Usually presumed to occur at cold temperatures, it can happen at an air temperature as high as 70°F, especially if the person is wet from rain or sweat and/or the conditions are windy. Since temperatures on the Mt. Whitney Trail between Trail Camp and the summit rarely rise above 70°F, hypothermia is a condition to take seriously when planning your hike. Hypothermia can occur with little warning and rapidly leads to a loss of mental function, which is why you must be aware of the early symptoms. You should constantly monitor yourself and group members for symptoms of hypothermia if attempting the summit on a cold, wet, or windy day. It is because of these very real dangers that you should carry extra clothes and a space blanket up the mountain.

Hypothermia sets in when the core body temperature drops below 95°F, only a 3.6°F decrease from normal. The first symptom is shivering—the body's attempt to rewarm itself. Signs of confusion and difficulty speaking may occur when the core temperature drops below 94°F. In the advanced stages of hypothermia, shivering stops, the body's core temperature drops below 90°F, and a person may no longer feel cold. He or she will become incoherent, with severely limited judgment. Death can result if your body temperature drops below 80°F.

Mild hypothermia can be treated in the field, while severe hypothermia must to be treated in a medical facility so the patient can be rewarmed properly. Poor heart function and sudden cardiac death is possible if a severely hypothermic patient is not handled carefully.

This makes it imperative to catch and reverse mild hypothermia before the condition worsens.

If an injury (or poor planning) forces you to spend a night on the mountain, if your clothes get wet in a storm, or if you are under-dressed on a cold, windy day, you are at severe risk of hypother-mia. Here are a few ways to minimize your chances of becoming hypothermic:

- Wear a hat. A large proportion of heat loss is through the head.
- If you end up with wet clothes, change into dry clothes immediately.
- If you are waiting for group members and find yourself get-ting cold, put on extra clothes, move out of the wind, and pace back and forth, swinging arms and legs vigorously to enhance circulation.
- If you are forced to spend a night on the mountain, find a sheltered location out of the wind, and huddle together with other group members, minimizing the surface area exposed to the cold conditions.

If you suspect someone in your group is hypothermic:

- Get the individual into a location sheltered from the wind.
- Make sure the person is wearing warm, dry clothes.
- If the patient is conscious and can swallow, feed the person warm, sweet liquids or easily digested foods.
- If someone is carrying a sleeping bag, the hypothermic per-son should be put in a pre-warmed sleeping bag, with warm water bottles placed inside.
- Monitor the patient's pulse and breathing, and body temper-ature, if possible. Plan for an evacuation if the patient does not improve. If the condition is severe, get help immediately. Also remember that severely hypothermic patients may appear to lack a pulse, but that does not mean the person is deceased.

Hydration

Dehydration is yet another ailment that leads to headaches and low energy. The body needs to maintain a constant amount of water in its cells and tissues to function, as well as to effectively transport blood and oxygen to the organs. While hiking, you will lose water by urinating, by sweating, and during respiration. The latter can be greatly exacerbated at high altitude, because you breathe more rapidly and the air is very dry.

However, it is also unhealthy to drink too much water, which can upset the balance of electrolytes in your body. You must keep up with water loss, but do not overdo it. Some references suggest you drink 24 ounces of water per hour while walking—an amount that could lead you to consume 13.5 quarts during an 18-hour day. This

WATERBORNE PESTS

Unless you plan to carry all the water you need for your hike (approximately 5 to 9 quarts), you'll need to obtain water on the trail. The southern fork of Lone Pine Creek sees such heavy use that most hikers choose to treat water along the Mt. Whitney Trail to prevent contamination with protozoa like giardia or cryptosporidium or bacteria like E. coli. However, you are unlikely to contract a virus from water in the Sierra Nevada; viruses do not survive long in the cold, harsh conditions of the alpine environment.

If you choose not to treat your water, there are several sources that, until they intersect the Mt. Whitney Trail, do not pass through heavily used areas. They include a spring in Bighorn Park, east of Outpost Camp; the outlet from Mirror Lake; and the spring that appears about 400 feet above Trail Camp. (See articles by Dr. Robert Derlet and Dr. Robert Rockwell in the Yosemite Association's "Nature Notes" archive for additional information on the purity of Sierra water sources: www.yosemite.org/naturenotes/archive.htm.)

If you do choose to treat your water, keep in mind that different treatment methods kill or remove different microbes:

- **Chemical purification (e.g. iodine or chlorine):** This is the easiest method of treating water—simply

is not realistic for most people and possibly not healthy du€
electrolyte depletion (see the section on fuel, page 44). Indeed, €
under much hotter desert conditions, 8 quarts per day is generally
adequate, and 5 to 9 quarts during a one-day ascent of Mt. Whitney
(or nearly twice as much during a two-day ascent) should suffice for
most people.

Initial signs of dehydration include thirst, a dry mouth, fatigue, dark
urine, dry skin, and loss of appetite. As the condition worsens, you
may note nausea, headaches, muscle cramps, increased respiration
and heart rate, and decreased sweating and urination. If a member
of your group gets dehydrated, have that person take a break and
slowly drink water with electrolytes. Severe dehydration requires
medical attention.

add drops or a tablet—but you have to wait about
20 minutes to drink your water, which will be left
with a distinct chemical flavor. In addition, chemical
purification might not kill cryptosporidium, so if this
microbe becomes more common in the Sierra, this
method will no longer be practical.

- **Water filter:** Water filters should remove all bacteria
  and protozoa, but the pores are too large to remove
  viruses. The advantages of filtering are that it
  removes all microorganisms of concern (in the Sierra
  Nevada) and doesn't leave a flavor in your water. But
  it can be time-consuming to filter water. If you are
  part of a large group with a single water filter, make
  sure the filter is in continuous use during your break,
  because you can lose a lot of time if many people
  need to filter right when you want to start walking.
- **Ultraviolet light purifier (e.g. SteriPEN):**Ultraviolet
  light damages the DNA of all microorganisms, ren-
  dering them harmless. Water must be clear for the
  ultraviolet light to function, so water with silt must
  be filtered.
- **Boiling:** Boiling kills all microorganisms, but is very
  time-consuming, requires a stove and fuel, and is
  not practical for dayhikers.

Food

You will burn approximately 6000 calories during your one-day ascent of Mt. Whitney and about 9000 calories during a two-day journey. Although you're unlikely to consume that many calories on your walk, don't skimp on food to save weight.

Food provides the body with the molecules the cells—including the cells in the muscles—use as energy. Food is also the body's source of various ions, or electrolytes. It's important to eat frequently as you exert yourself, because your muscle cells will run out of glycogen, the form in which they store carbohydrates.

"Electrolytes" is a catchall term for a collection of salts, including sodium, potassium, and calcium; the relative concentrations of these electrolytes is essential in maintaining nerve and muscle

POOR METABOLIC FUNCTION

Metabolism is the sum of all the chemical and physical processes that occur in the body that turn the food you eat and the oxygen you breathe into energy that the body can use. These processes occur within the cells, and poor metabolic function can happen if there is an insufficient supply of food and oxygen to the cells, or if the cells are not effectively using the food and oxygen they receive.

The link between high elevation and hypoxia, a deficiency in the amount of oxygen reaching the body's tissues, is obvious. However, other conditions, including dehydration, hypothermia, and electrolyte depletion also, by complex physiological pathways, cause poor metabolic function by affecting the supply of substances to the cells and the use of substances by the cells.

Since all of these conditions make cells less efficient at metabolizing food and oxygen, they physiologically reinforce one another, exacerbating the poor cellular function caused by other conditions. This means that if you are dehydrated or low on electrolytes, you are more likely to display symptoms associated with poor metabolic function. For instance, headaches at high elevation are generally attributed to altitude sickness. However, they are probably due, in part, to dehydration and not eating enough.

function, blood acidity, hydration, and the delivery of oxygen to your cells.

While your kidneys do a good job balancing the relative concentrations of the different electrolytes, they can do their job only if the electrolytes are present in your body. It's up to you to consume sufficient food. As you hike, stop frequently and eat small amounts of food. If it's a hot day and you are sweating a lot, it is a good idea to supplement the electrolytes (and sugars) in your food with electrolyte-containing energy drinks. Also be sure to drink electrolyte mixes if your appetite is diminished due to the altitude and exertion. Finally, beware of drinking too much water, which can throw off your electrolyte balance, especially if you're not eating adequately.

HINT: I prefer the flavor of plain water while hiking, so instead of filling a whole bottle with an energy drink, I bring a small cup and bag of electrolyte mix and mix up a cup during a few of my longer breaks.

Lightning

From the upper switchbacks to the east of Trail Crest all the way to the summit of Mt. Whitney, the trail is exposed, leaving hikers vulnerable to lightning strikes. Moreover, should a storm suddenly develop, there is no escape route along these last miles. Byrd Surby, the first recorded fatality on Mt. Whitney, was killed by lightning near the summit in 1904, just eight days after the Mt. Whitney Trail was completed. Lightning on or near the summit has actually killed very few people, but more have been struck and sustained injuries of varying severity.

As described in the weather section on page 31, thunderstorms are much rarer in the Sierra Nevada than in most other mountain ranges, and it is often safe to be at high elevations throughout the day. However, on other days, it is imperative that you head down by noon.

Before you begin your hike, check the weather forecast at the National Oceanic and Atmospheric Administration website: Go to www.wrh.noaa.gov/vef, and click on a location due south of Bishop and a bit north of the latitude of Death Valley. If the probability of precipitation is 10 percent, it is my experience that you will stay dry 50 percent of the time, but you need to get a very early start to safely summit Mt. Whitney. If the probability of precipitation is even 20 percent, you will probably get wet and should accept from the outset that you may not be able to summit.

Regardless of the forecast, turn around promptly when you see tall, dark, flat-bottomed cumulonimbus (thunder) clouds nearby. Clouds can build very quickly: Scattered white clouds can evolve into a nasty storm in less than two hours, less time than it takes most people to hike round-trip from Trail Crest to the summit. It takes even less time for a seemingly distant storm to move overhead. If you hear even distant thunder, head down quickly. In clear air, thunder can be heard from a distance of approximately 10 miles. (While lightning can move vertically through the sky and can strike while there is clear sky above, this is rare and is not a major concern.)

Lightning occurs to alleviate charge imbalances between the clouds (usually negative) and the ground (usually positive). These imbalances develop because negative and positive charges are separated within clouds, leading to charged water molecules. The negative charges within a thundercloud cause equal positive charges to develop on the ground. Negatively charged "leaders" descend from the cloud and can lead to a much stronger return strike if they drop to within 100 feet of the ground. Most lightning strikes occur at the beginning and at the end of a thunderstorm. Also, you generally have a brief "safe" period to move after a nearby lightning strike, before the ground charges redevelop.

PROTECTING YOURSELF AGAINST LIGHTNING

In 1990, after a lightning-caused fatality in the summit hut (and a subsequent lawsuit), the hut was retrofitted. It was grounded with wires and a wood floor was installed to insulate visitors from the ground. Nonetheless, it is still recommended that you do not sit out an electric storm inside the hut. Instead, should you be caught near the summit in a lightning storm, follow the tips described here to help minimize your chances of being struck and to reduce the risk of sustaining severe injury if you are struck. Once a storm is overhead, it is more important to follow these rules than to try to reach lower ground:

- Get in the lightning position, both to reduce the likelihood of a direct strike and to reduce the seriousness of injury you are likely to sustain. The National Outdoor Leadership School recommends squatting or sitting as low as possible and wrapping your arms around your legs. This position minimizes your body's surface area, so there's less of a chance for a ground current to flow through you. Close your eyes, and keep your feet together to prevent the current from flowing in one foot and out the other.

- Squat on top of an insulated pad or a pile of clothes, if available.
- Place any metal objects and wet ropes at least 50 feet from you, as they can conduct the current, leading to greater injury. (This probably includes your backpack.)
- If you are stuck in flattish terrain above treeline, crouch on top of a rock (but not the highest one, of course) that is somewhat elevated or otherwise detached from the rocks underneath it.
- Stay out of shallow caves and away from overhangs.
- If you are part of a larger group, people should be at least 50 feet apart, so multiple people are not injured by a single strike.
- Sit in an area where you are less than 50 feet from, but not directly next to, a much taller object such as a tree.
- Although it's not much of an issue high on the Mt. Whitney Trail, avoid individual trees and the tallest trees, instead seeking a larger grove. Also, remember that if a tree is struck, the lightning can discharge through the roots, so stay a good distance away from large trees.

TREATING LIGHTNING INJURIES

Should a member of your party be struck by lightning and stop breathing, immediately begin CPR. CPR is more likely to be successful following a lightning strike than many other injuries, as the electrical shock can stop a person's heart from beating without actually causing much internal damage. Indeed, 80 percent of strikes are not fatal. (But be prepared to continue CPR or rescue breathing for a long period of time.)

Treat burns by immersing small wounds in cool water (or if available, run cool water over the wound), applying antibiotic ointment to the wound, and covering it with a sterile gauze pad held in place with tape. Plan evacuation and seek medical attention immediately.

For more information about lightning safety, look for the guidelines produced by the National Outdoor Leadership School at www.nols. edu.

Falling and Knee Problems

A common ailment on the Mt. Whitney Trail is knee problems, especially during the steep descent. Don't be tempted to run down the trail for an earlier dinner or because you continued to the summit after your turnaround time: Most injuries occur at the end of the day, when you're tired.

The two best ways to avoid knee problems are to walk slowly and to use trekking poles. Walking slowly puts less force on your knee with each step, and using trekking poles takes some weight off your knees. And a bizarre suggestion: Especially if you're wearing a heavy pack, turn around to walk down those occasional really tall steps backward, which significantly reduces the pressure on your knees by employing the stronger muscles of your upper legs. While I can't tell you how much this reduces strain on your knees, it helps me tremendously, and I have converted many friends. Also, if you have knee problems, wear a knee brace.

If you do twist a knee, stop promptly and take anti-inflammatory drugs (such as ibuprofen or naproxen). You may choose to wrap your knee with the elastic bandage in your first-aid kit, but don't wrap it too tightly. Then continue (slowly!) down the hill, with the help of your group members and perhaps some trekking poles as crutches. (If you twist an ankle, using sports tape is better than using an elastic bandage, as the elastic bandage will provide less stability and support.)

Blisters

Even with broken-in, comfortable shoes, it is easy to get blisters when ascending (and descending) more than 6000 feet and hiking 21 miles. However, there are many tricks to minimize the severity of blisters and to tackle hot spots are soon as they begin to form. For instance:

- Wear the same shoes you wore on your training hikes (see the section on footwear, on page 69).

- Make sure you are wearing well-padded, dry socks. If you are especially prone to sweaty feet, bring along an extra pair of socks to switch into halfway up the climb.
- Cover potential hot spots with sports tape, another tape, or moleskin (see the first-aid kit section, on page 74), either before you start or as soon as you sense a hot spot forming. Use long enough pieces of tape so that they don't simply fall off your heel.

The book *Lightweight Backpacking and Camping* (Beartooth Mountain Press, 2005) has many suggestions for reducing the possibility of injuries, especially blisters. Preventative measures include treating your feet with alcohol for the week before a long hike to toughen your foot and applying Tuf-Skin to your feet before your walk.

If a blister should develop, treat it promptly. Some people are content taping over small blisters with a piece of sports tape, but it is often better to apply blister bandages or a piece of moleskin, followed by sports tape. An old trick is to cut a piece of moleskin into a donut shape, such that the blister is surrounded by a raised ring of moleskin, although many people now use blister bandages. Large blisters are best drained with a sterile pin before patching. Blisters on toes can be very difficult to treat, as taping one toe often causes a blister on the neighboring toe when the tape (or other blister treatment) rubs. Another option is to tape a toe blister with thin tape to minimize rubbing and to proactively tape the neighboring toe.

Bears

The American black bears' taste for human food makes them a big nuisance along the Mt. Whitney Trail. But unless you're fighting them for your food, they are not a danger to humans. Despite their name, black bears come in a variety of colors, including tan and brown. As a result of human visits as well as human food in the high-elevation Sierra Nevada, these smart and highly adaptable creatures have expanded their range upward in these mountains. Historically found predominately in the mid-elevation conifer forests of the western Sierra, black bears now roam up to the Sierra Crest and along many of the eastern Sierra drainages, including Lone Pine Creek.

During the 1990s, hikers increasingly returned to trailheads with shreds of stuff sacks and food wrappers. As a result, hikers visiting many parts of the Sierra, including the Mt. Whitney Trail, are now required to carry bear-resistant food canisters (see page 79 for more information). Thankfully, the strict food-storage policies are working: At least 95 percent of hikers are complying with the regulations, very few people are losing food, and, in some locations, bears appear to be retreating to lower elevations. When camping, make sure your food is always by your side during the day, and lock your food canister promptly when you finish preparing your meals. This is especially important at Trail Camp, where you will find quite aggressive marmots and ravens, and they aren't about to relocate to lower elevations.

PREVENTING COMMON TRAIL HAZARDS

Hazard	Prevention
Altitude sickness	• Drink plenty of water and eat food. • Take acclimation hikes.
Hypothermia	• Carry all your warm clothes and a space blanket to the top of the mountain.
Dehydration	• Drink 5 to 9 quarts of water during your ascent.
Low energy/ fatigue	• Eat small snacks every few hours. • Add electrolyte solution to your water.
Lightning	• Do not attempt to summit if there are thunderheads nearby.
Knee injuries	• Use trekking poles. • Go slowly.
Blisters	• Wear broken-in, sturdy shoes or boots. • Apply sports tape to potential hot spots before the hike. • Stop and patch hot spots as soon as you feel them.
Bears	• Store food in a bear-resistant canister.

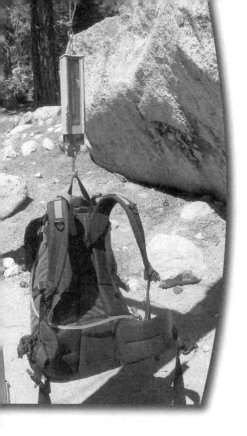

☙ *3* ❧
Preparations and Planning

Once you have decided to climb Mt. Whitney, it's time to start planning. The Mt. Whitney Trail, or more properly, the subset of the trail within the Whitney Zone, is currently the only location in the Sierra Nevada that imposes a quota on dayhikers. In addition, like nearly every trailhead in the Sierra, quotas limit the number of backpackers departing from the Whitney Portal trailhead. The implementation of the day-use quota in 1996 was an excellent move: On my first ascent, in mid-September 1995, I reached the summit before 9:30 AM, and there were already 30 people vying for the best vista points on the summit. By noon, there were approximately 200 people crowding the area. So many people led to resource damage and detracted enormously from each person's wilderness experience. The number of people on the trail certainly disturbed me and I avoided the summit for several years. It is still a busy trail, but thanks to the quotas, which limit the number of hikers to 100 dayhikers and 60 backpackers, there are few enough people on the trail that you actually begin to recognize (and greet) people as the hike progresses. (Beginning in 2008, the dayhike quota included permits obtained by dayhikers ascending the use-trail up

Above: Weighing a pack at Whitney Portal

51

the North Fork of Lone Pine Creek to the technical routes on Mt. Whitney—further diminishing the number of people on the Mt. Whitney Trail.) The downside is that hiking Mt. Whitney cannot be a spur-of-the-moment decision, as you need to choose whether you want to dayhike or backpack, as well as your preferred hiking dates, by February 1, the date when the permit lottery opens for the season.

Dayhike vs. Overnight

Some people enjoy attempting the summit in a single, 21-mile day, while others prefer to spread their ascent over two, three, or more days. While many factors may influence your decision, the debate usually comes down whether you want to put in the extra effort required to carry overnight gear for the pleasure of a more relaxing ascent and a backcountry camping experience.

Here are some reasons to dayhike:

- You dislike carrying an overnight pack.
- Permits are easier to obtain for a dayhike, especially if you have limited choices of dates.
- You prefer the faster walking pace possible with only a daypack on your back.

And some reasons to do an overnight trip:

- You prefer the more leisurely pace associated with backpacking.
- You enjoy spending a night in the middle of the mountains.
- You want the extra night(s) to acclimatize at an intermediate elevation before pushing for the summit.
- You know your legs and feet do not wish to travel 21 miles in a single day.

I've summited Mt. Whitney, and many other peaks, both as long dayhikes and as part of a backpacking trip, and the experiences are completely different. On a backpacking trip, the camaraderie of my climbing partners and the time spent together in camp are important parts of the excursion. I tend to spend more time enjoying my surroundings and really appreciate that I am in the middle of an amazing wilderness area. On a long dayhike, I focus more on the physical requirements of getting up and down the mountain safely, knowing I will be exhausted by the end of the day, but also keeping in mind I must make it back to the car by dark. I enjoy the physical and mental challenges that come with pushing myself hard, but there is decidedly less "wilderness experience" in my trip. A backpacking trip along the Mt. Whitney Trail merges a bit of both experiences, since summiting a tall peak is still the goal of the trip. But a dayhike accentuates the endurance aspects of the hike.

When to Go

Like most people hiking the Mt. Whitney Trail, you probably care most about maximizing your chances of summiting. This means you should pick a time of year when the hike requires the least physical and mental exertion and has the lowest likelihood of bad weather. This is a probability game, since you can't shift your summit date by a week to match the weather forecast. In the Sierra Nevada, the absolute best conditions generally exist during July and August. However, we are blessed with a long summer, and most days between June and September are pleasant on the mountain.

Factors that might influence your preferred summit date include:

- **Snow on the trail:** Your first consideration should be to pick a date after most snow has melted—early to mid-July is a safe bet most years. Slogging through residual snow on the trail, especially on the 99 switchbacks above Trail Camp, is very tiring. Your feet slip around with each step, and if the day is warm, you will posthole (sink into the snow). In addition, you are more likely to get blisters if your feet get wet.
- **Thunderstorms:** Most thunderstorms occur in late July and August, but they can also occur during June, early July, and September.
- **Strong winds:** Powerful winds, which are more common in June and September than in midsummer, will sap your energy.
- **Temperature:** The warmest days are in mid- to late July.
- **Pacific storms:** Weak Pacific storms are often still blowing through in early June, and they return by early to mid-September. The late spring and early fall storms usually drop little precipitation but are very blustery and cold for 12 to 24 hours while they pass.
- **Day length:** As long as you are content to walk up much of the mountain in the dark, this is not a major consideration, but days start getting shorter much more rapidly in

mid-August. (I prefer starting in the dark and enjoying the alpenglow on the peaks once I am already above Mirror Lake.)

- **The moon cycle:** A few days after a full moon is the best time for early-morning walking, because the moon will not set until after the sun rises. A few days before a full moon is my favorite time for backpacking, because evenings are moonlit. For some people, summiting at dawn on the day of the full moon and simultaneously watching moonset and sunrise is well worth the effort of hiking 10.5 miles in the dark.

- **Air quality:** Forest fires around the Sierra (and beyond) can result in a perpetual haze in the Sierra during midsummer. The clarity tends to increase following the first small Pacific front to blow through in September.

Wilderness Permits

The most likely stumbling point during the planning stage is getting a permit to enter the Mt. Whitney Zone. (Note: This information pertains only to the Mt. Whitney Trail; certain regulations are different for other trails in the region.)

HINT: If you miss the lottery but can arrange your schedule to do a midweek dayhike, there is a very good chance there will be unclaimed permits. These are available at noon the day before your intended hike—and they're free. Many days, there are 20 unclaimed permits, but you must be at the Eastern Sierra InterAgency Visitor Center outside of Lone Pine at noon the day before you wish to hike to take advantage of these.

Permits are required for both dayhikes and overnight backpacking trips, and trailhead quotas are in effect from May 1 to November 1. To request a permit, you must enter the permit lottery by submitting an application by mail sometime during the month of February. (Permits postmarked earlier in February have an advantage over those submitted at the end of the month.) There are no first-come, first-served permits available, and only occasionally can you get a permit if someone cancels (see "Hint," left). The maximum group size for a permit is 15.

To submit your application, download a form from www.fs.fed.us/r5/inyo/recreation/wild/whitneylottery.shtml, fill it out, and mail the form, as well as a $15 per-person check, to Inyo National Forest:

Inyo National Forest Wilderness Permit Offices
351 Pacu Lane, Suite 200
Bishop, California 93514
760-873-2485 (Wilderness Information)

There are a few quirky rules to the permit process:

- Since permits are not transferable, list alternate leaders on your permit application if you want to make sure your group can still use the permit if the original "leader" is unable to go on the trip.
- You cannot apply for permits for two successive days. If you wish to do a moonlight ascent, you must reach the Mt. Whitney Zone boundary no earlier than midnight—or cheat by a few hours and assume the rangers aren't also doing a moonlight ascent.
- If you wish to do a longer backpacking trip, you can hike in at a different trailhead, such as Cottonwood Pass, New Army Pass, or Kearsarge Pass, and have an easier time obtaining a permit. See other Wilderness Press books, including *Sierra South*, *Sequoia National Park*, and *John Muir Trail* for details on doing this.

You will be notified by mail that you have received your permit, and if you don't get a permit, the agency will return your check. However, if you get a permit for dates that you cannot make, you will not get your money back.

To pick up your wilderness permit, you must go to the Eastern Sierra InterAgency Visitor Center (760-876-6222), located 2 miles south of the center of Lone Pine, at the southeast corner of the intersection of Hwy. 395 and State Rte. 136. Overnight permits must be picked up or confirmed by 10 AM on the departure date. Dayhike permits must be picked up or confirmed by noon the day *before* the permit date. To confirm your permit, call the Inyo National Forest Wilderness Permit Reservation Office at 760-873-2483. If you wish to pick up your permit after hours, call the number above and have your permit left in the night box, located in a small kiosk along State Rte. 136. For additional information on Mt. Whitney Zone permits, see www.fs.fed.us/r5/inyo/recreation/wild/mtwhitney.shtml.

HINT: To better your chances of getting a Whitney Zone permit:

- *Get your permit reservation in the mail on February 1.*
- *Include many possible dates.*
- *Include midweek options.*

Training

Hiking 21 miles is a major undertaking (especially if you choose to do it in a day), and climbing well over 6000 feet requires a lot of effort. Long before you start worrying about acclimatizing to high elevation (see below), you need to get used to walking long distances up and down hills. In other words, you need to be in relatively good aerobic shape, have toned the needed muscles, and have excellent endurance. You do not need to be fast.

Any aerobic exercise will help you get in shape, but the muscles used extensively for walking up and down hills can really only be conditioned by walking up and down hills. If you live somewhere with hills, the best form of training is, unsurprisingly, to take long walks. However, if your surroundings are flatter, or you don't have time to hike hills regularly, cities are full of training opportunities: walk up and down staircases in a tall building, walk up and down bleachers in a local stadium, or use a stair machine at a gym. Do not underestimate the descent; this long downhill section catches many people unprepared. Also, knee injuries are more likely if the muscles you need to descend gracefully are not strong.

Testing your endurance ahead of time is important in ensuring that you are physically and mentally ready to walk for many hours. If you can do a fast-paced 10- to 12-mile hike in hilly terrain, your physical capabilities are unlikely to limit your success. For many newcomers to hiking (or other endurance sports), the mental game is equally difficult. You need to know how to keep going once you are tired—such as on the way back down, when you've reached your goal and the car is still 10.5 miles away. Successfully finishing training walks and other workouts, even if you are tired or bored, is one good way to know you are ready for Mt. Whitney.

The final reason for training hikes is to break in a pair of hiking boots or shoes (see more on footwear on page 69). You are more likely to succeed on summit day if painful feet aren't stopping you.

ACCLIMATION HIKES

The final stage in your training for Mt. Whitney is to get your body acclimatized to higher elevations. It is best if you can spend several days hiking at moderate elevations just before attempting Mt. Whitney. However, I also recommend that you spend at least one weekend during the previous month (or months) hiking above

10,000 feet. Indeed, research has shown that repeated exposure high elevations can help you prepare for a tall summit, even if it i immediately before your climb.

If you live in northern California, a weekend trip to the Tahoe area, the Tuolumne Meadows section of Yosemite, or anywhere in between provides ample hiking options. If you live in southern California, 11,502-foot Mt. San Gorgonio, 10,834-foot San Jacinto Peak, and 10,064-foot Mt. San Antonio (a.k.a. Mt. Baldy), are good acclimation hikes.

In addition to acclimation hikes you take over the previous month, it is best to do one or more high-elevation hikes within two days of attempting the mountain, especially if you will be dayhiking Mt. Whitney. Three possibilities near Whitney Portal are: the trail to Trail Pass from the Cottonwood Pass parking area, the Cottonwood Lakes Trail to the Cottonwood Lakes Basin, and the trail from Onion Valley toward Kearsarge Pass. Remember, your goal is to acclimate your body, not to tire your legs or bash your feet. A 1000- to 2000-foot climb and a 5- to 8-mile day is all you should do the day before you head up the Mt. Whitney Trail, and you may choose to do only a portion of one of the hikes described below. If you decide to hike up a trail not listed here, select a trailhead between 8000 and 10,000 feet—not too high, not too low.

HIKE 1

Cottonwood Pass Trailhead to Trail Pass and Beyond

Distance: 7.4 miles out and back

Elevation: ± 1200 feet

Maps: Tom Harrison *Golden Trout Wilderness Trail*, USGS 7.5-minute *Cirque Peak*

Overview: This short walk leads you through exquisite fox-tail pine forests as you climb to Trail Pass and then follow the Pacific Crest Trail south toward Mulkey Pass.

How to Get There: From Lone Pine, drive 3.5 miles west along the Whitney Portal Road and then turn left onto the Horseshoe Meadow Road. Continue straight ahead approximately 20 miles until you reach the end of the road, the Cottonwood Pass Trailhead.

Leaving the Cottonwood Pass Trailhead, head west to skirt the northern edge of Horseshoe Meadow. After 0.3 mile, you reach a junction and turn left (south), toward Trail Pass. Now crossing sandy mounds characteristic of open flats in the southern Sierra, you cross a stream and climb slightly into foxtail pine forest. The trail climbs gently as it circles around the head of the smaller Round Valley meadow, and then begins switchbacking to Trail Pass. This stretch of trail is through beautiful forest of foxtail pines, whose needles encircle the tips of the branches, giving them the appearance of bottlebrushes. As you climb higher, the trees have ever more character after a lifetime of being bashed by winter winds.

After 1.9 miles and a 600-foot climb, you reach Trail Pass and a junction with the Pacific Crest Trail (PCT). You can now follow the PCT in either direction for as long (or short) as you wish. I recommend heading south (left), where you will be treated to sporadic views of the Kern Plateau, with its expansive meadows separated by

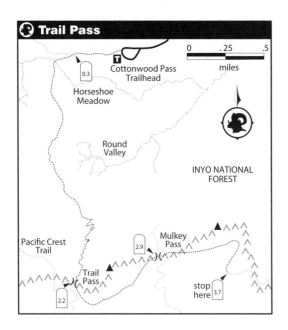

craggy granite outcrops and perfectly round cinder cones. After 0.7 mile, you reach Mulkey Pass, at which point you will cross another (less well-maintained) trail leading from Horseshoe Meadow. Another 0.8 mile leads you up to a collection of granite outcrops dotted with exquisite, weather-beaten trees. This is a good vista, and a nice place to have lunch and turn around.

HIKE 2   Cottonwood Lakes Trailhead to Cottonwood Lakes Basin

Distance: 9.6 miles out and back to Cottonwood Lakes

Elevation: ± 1100 feet to Cottonwood Lakes

Maps: Tom Harrison *Golden Trout Wilderness Trail*, USGS 7.5-minute *Cirque Peak*

Overview: This is a lovely trail to walk, for although it starts high, it climbs just slightly more than 1000 feet to reach the Cottonwood Lakes, an easy walk through forest and open meadows.

How to Get There: From Lone Pine, drive 3.5 miles west along the Whitney Portal Road, and then turn left onto the Horseshoe Meadows Road. Continue 20 miles until you reach signs pointing you right, toward the trail to Cottonwood Lakes and New Army Pass. Take the right-hand fork, and follow the road, which climbs slightly. Pass a turnoff to the local pack station, and continue to the hikers' parking lot near a pair of campgrounds.

The trailhead is located at the northwestern edge of the parking lot, next to the large information board and the toilets. The trail heads west from this point. (Note that some 7.5-minute USGS maps do not accurately portray the configuration of the trailhead or the beginning of this trail.) The first miles of this trail are nearly flat, passing alternately through stands of lodgepole pine and foxtail pine. The former prefers the flatter, more sheltered terrain, while the foxtails thrive on the more exposed, sandy, dry slopes.

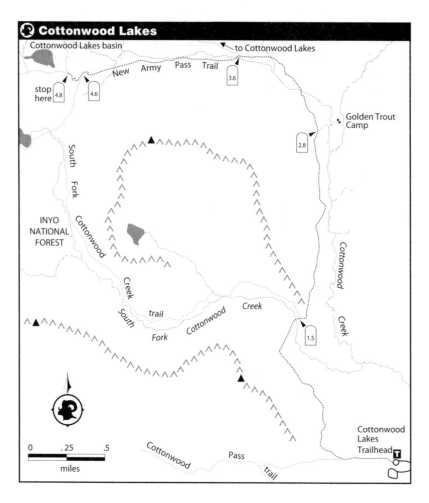

The trail continues through the forest, crosses the South Fork of Cottonwood Creek, and after 2.8 reaches an unsigned junction (stay left) for the Golden Trout Camp before a large meadow.

Shortly after the junction for the Golden Trout Camp you enter John Muir Wilderness. Beyond the Golden Trout Camp, the trail trends to the left, passes through another meadow, and begins a steeper climb to the Cottonwood Lakes basin. Soon thereafter, the trail bends nearly due west, and follows this trajectory up to and through the Cottonwood Lakes basin.

Stay left at a junction labeled Cottonwood Lakes, right at the junction to the South Fork lakes (at 11,000 feet), and, just beyond a third junction, you reach the first of the Cottonwood Lakes, 2.0 miles after the wilderness boundary. Stop here and enjoy lunch along the banks of this lake. Unlike in most of the High Sierra, trout are native to the Cottonwood Lakes basin. As a result, special fishing regulations are in place to protect the local populations of golden trout.

HIKE 3 Onion Valley Trailhead toward Kearsarge Pass

Distance: 7.8 miles out and back to the plateau below Kearsarge Pass

Elevation: ± 2000

Maps: Tom Harrison *Kings Canyon High Country Trail*; USGS 7.5-minute *Kearsarge Peak*

Overview: The trail to Kearsarge Pass skirts several lakes that are popular fishing locations and campsites, and then it climbs to timberline for a vista of craggy ridges.

How to Get There: From Lone Pine, drive 15 miles north along Hwy. 395 to the town of Independence. From the center of Independence take Market Street (Onion Valley Road) 12.5 miles westward to its terminus at the Onion Valley Trailhead.

Several trails depart from this large parking area, and the Kearsarge Pass Trail is due west, beyond the toilets and the cluster of bear-boxes. From the edge of the parking area, you climb an open slope dotted with dry site shrubs, including sagebrush. Except for a brief interlude beneath tall red firs, the trail continues through similar vegetation for 1.5 miles. Throughout this section, there are views down-canyon to the parking area and beyond.

The trail then skirts above Little Pothole Lake, passing through a few stretches of moister vegetation. After another 0.7 mile, you reach the outlet of Gilbert Lake, around which there are several campsites. The next section of trail passes through a lodgepole pine forest, providing welcome shade.

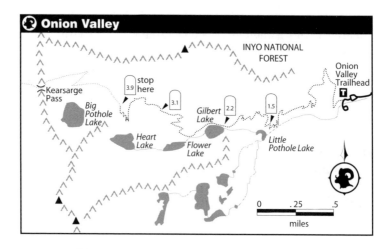

A short distance beyond Gilbert Lake, you spy Flower Lake, another lovely picnic location, to the left of the trail. The trail now turns away from the drainage, switchbacking up the slope to the north. Approximately 0.9 mile beyond Gilbert Lake, the trail emerges from the forest in a little subalpine flat. Bright pink Sierra primroses are common beneath boulders along this section. Steep talus slopes loom above you as the trail bends left and skirts across a barren slope, leading to a series of tight switchbacks up a slope dotted with stunted whitebark pines. Far below, Heart Lake is visible, accessible via the inlet to Flower Lake.

After another 0.8 mile, the grade lessens—a good turnaround spot, as you have now hiked 3.9 miles and climbed 2000 feet. The trail continues up an increasingly steep slope of sand, gravel, and the occasional boulder to Kearsarge Pass. Switchbacks are visible all the way to the top of the pass, somewhat to the right of the ridge's low point.

Considerations for Summiting

By the time you reach Whitney Portal, you will have spent many hours planning, training, and assembling your pack of summit gear. This section covers a few more considerations for your trip: group dynamics, pace, and breaks. These are topics to read about before you leave home and to have firmly etched in your mind during your hike. For each of these, I can provide advice, but no tangible "rules," because how you implement my suggestions is affected by individualistic factors: what pace and break schedule works best for you, and your judgment and attitudes about pushing yourself, safety, and group etiquette.

GROUP DYNAMICS

If you will be ascending Mt. Whitney as part of a group, it is important to know each other's expectations before you begin your hike. Realizing partway up the mountain that you have different criteria for turning around, different paces, or simply different goals for the excursion can easily lead to bad feelings and a disappointing hike—not to mention an unsuccessful summit bid. You should discuss these factors thoroughly and honestly with all potential hiking companions.

In my experience, the single greatest source of problems between group members has been neglecting to communicate before reaching the trailhead about levels of experience and goals for the trip. On a trip to 14,370-foot Mt. Williamson, someone assured me he had experience at high altitude, only to explain later that he had only once been to 10,000 feet. On many trips, people have indicated they do not mind hiking by themselves if the group should wish to continue faster. But often it turns out that they expressed that opinion only because they wished to join a trip, not because they were actually comfortable hiking alone. On the trip itself, they become resentful if the group continues ahead without them.

However, most trips run smoothly. Usually the group remains together, with the faster hikers taking more time to take in their surroundings and the slower hikers feeling a bit pushed, but not dreadfully so. This works because all group members make small compromises and all have the same timeline and agenda in mind.

Also bear in mind that hiking as part of a group will probably cause the entire group to ascend a bit more slowly, because each person will be slowest at a different point in time. However, it also tends to be a lot more fun to have friends with whom to share the experience than to pound up the trail on your own.

Nearly every hiking team—unless you are accompanying a few friends whose pace you know—will be comprised of people with different hiking speeds. This requires compromises, patience, and understanding by everyone as you figure out how to accommodate the pace of different group members. Slower hikers may feel bad for holding up the group, and therefore agree to turn around even though they would very much like to summit. If the group has agreed in advance to take a certain amount of time for the hike and remain as a group, and you are still within that timetable, the group should stick together. Encourage the slower person to keep going and take some weight from his/her pack. In contrast, a hiker who cannot keep up the designated pace should realize this fact, and agree to wait, alone or with a friend, while others continue to the summit. Because there is a trail to the top and there are many other people on the trail, it is usually even safe to hike on your own if the weather is good and it is not late in the day.

If you are part of a particularly large group, people are likely to spread out a little as the hike progresses; pick a "buddy" in advance, and stick with that person as you hike. A group of more than four or six may even agree to reassemble only at the summit—a big group generally has considerable inertia, as each person is likely to slow down the group at different times.

If the decision is made for the group to split, make sure everyone has agreed where the group will reassemble, whether it is at the car or somewhere up the trail. It is very important that everyone knows exactly where and when the meeting location is: Many a trip has turned sour when different people are waiting at different locations and cannot find their friends.

Some of the following questions will help you determine important concerns (if any) in your group's dynamics:

- Do group members think it is necessary to stick together, or can each person go at his or her own pace? While it is easiest to hike with people with similar paces, this rarely occurs. As described on page 66, most people have the best endurance when they hike at their preferred pace, neither too fast nor too slow. A good strategy is to allow people to pace them- selves, but to regroup every mile or two at a predesignated break spot. However, group members should always stick together in the dark or in bad weather.
- Do you plan to stick with a strict turnaround time? If the answer is yes, as it should be, decide on a timetable in advance (see page 100 for likely travel times) and agree to turn around at the whatever time you should have reached the summit. Since many mountaineering problems arise on the way down, especially if you are faced with waning

daylight, you should never continue upward after a predetermined turnaround time.

- Under what weather conditions would each person prefer to turn around? People differ in the amount of risk they are willing to tolerate when seeking the summit. No one should feel obliged to continue to the summit if they think conditions are risky—or particularly unpleasant. If you are the gung-ho person, you should continue to the summit on your own only if it is not late in the day and there are not whiteout conditions.

- Does everyone have the goal of summiting Mt. Whitney? If a group member is just coming to take a nice hike, never intending to continue past Trail Camp, he or she should express that in advance, since that person will be less inclined to take short breaks and forgo photo stops to stick to a timetable.

- Is one person the "group leader," calling the shots, or are you hiking as a cooperative, where a consensus must be reached for each decision? The advantage of reaching a group resolution is that everyone's interests have been discussed and no one feels disenfranchised. However, everyone's preference is unlikely to be accommodated and much time can be spent discussing the relative importance of each person's viewpoint. If there is a group leader, that person must listen to everyone's input and attempt to make a fair decision. I generally find that if the group leader is considerate—and that person is one of the most experienced hikers in the group—this leads to faster and often fairer decisions. A good group leader will take into account everyone's needs, even those of less vocal participants who might otherwise be ignored.

As you discuss these considerations, start to develop a plan for your hike. Make sure everyone has agreed upon a starting time, whether from Whitney Portal or a campsite along the trail. Nothing sets a day off to a worse start than pacing around at 4 AM, waiting for someone who hasn't yet gotten around to filling water bottles, taping heels, and the many other "quick" tasks that expand into a half-hour (or longer) delay. If you know you are slow in the morning, get organized the night before and wake up extra early.

PACE

One key to successfully completing a long hike is determining the pace that allows you to continue for the longest distance before your legs tire. The more practice hikes you take, especially at moderately high elevations, the better you will learn what pace gives you the best endurance. I have learned that I have a bit of a range of paces that feel "good" to my body, but if I have to move more quickly, I need far too many breaks and my legs get tired prematurely. Alternately, if I hike more slowly than my normal pace, my legs and breathing never settle into a sustainable rhythm, and both my endurance and motivation are much reduced.

In mountaineering, "slower and steady" wins the race—and that rule certainly applies to a hike up the Mt. Whitney Trail. As you ascend the mountain, keep reminding yourself that, regardless of your speed, having a slower, steady pace is preferable to moving in short, quick, bursts interrupted by breaks.

When hiking at high elevation, most people's pace is determined by their lung capacity for the first part of the walk, and—if they are acclimatized—by their legs toward the end of a long walk. If you find yourself continuously out of breath and needing frequent stops, slow down until your breaths and steps are in a steady, sustainable rhythm. It is difficult to find a pace to overcome tired legs; most people resort to short spurts and quick breaks to compensate for sore muscles. To avoid reaching this state too early, stretch before starting your walk, let your legs warm up during the first mile (see below), avoid too many long breaks on the way up, and keep eating food.

Observations and experience have taught me that most people start out too fast, even though it's advisable to start off more slowly. When you begin your hike, you need to give your muscles a chance to warm up and should therefore go more slowly than your "normal" pace for the first half mile to mile. On this trail, I force myself to move at about 70 percent of my normal pace until I cross the North Fork of Lone Pine Creek, 0.9 mile from the trailhead. At that point, I speed up a little, but I keep reminding myself that my legs have a long climb ahead and I need to walk slightly more slowly than I would on a shorter hike.

It's also advisable to slow down at high elevation. Between Trail Crest and the summit, much of which is fairly flat, people often

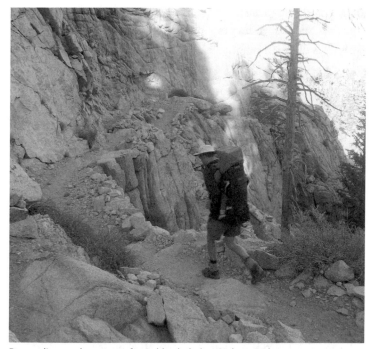

Descending an elegant set of switchbacks below Bighorn Park

attempt to hike along at a fast clip. With few exceptions, they stop every five (or fewer) minutes, exhausted and gasping for air. Meanwhile, slightly slower hikers walk by them during these breaks and inevitably reach the summit first. A good rule of thumb at high elevation is to keep slowing down until your lungs no longer determine your break schedule. This is, of course, an ideal that is difficult to reach, and even well-paced walkers will need to stop for 30-second quick breathers (see below) at the highest elevations.

BREAKS

As you are ascending Mt. Whitney, you will likely take many different sorts of breaks: 30-second breaks to catch your breath, especially on the switchbacks and the last miles to the summit, five- to 10-minute breaks to eat some food or patch blisters, and a couple longer breaks for a more substantial snack or lunch. No matter how well you pace yourself, everyone will end up taking lots of half-minute breathers—and quick drink breaks—especially at the highest elevations. Taking all these types of breaks is necessary, as they allow your body to recharge itself (and allow you to enjoy a quick conversation with your companions)—but don't dawdle beyond the suggested times, because you rapidly lose precious minutes.

You should plan on taking a five- to 10-minute break every one to two hours, making sure to eat snacks before your body feels low on energy. In addition, most groups will take one to two 20-minute breaks during the ascent and smart planners will schedule at least an hour for the summit. Be careful not to let short, half-minute breathers take up more than that; you don't want your leg muscles to cool down, and you don't want to lose the good walking rhythm you have established. Note that the suggested hiking times on page 100 assume that in addition to quick breathers, you take a 10-minute break for each hour on the trail, such that for a nine-hour ascent, you can take 90 minutes of breaks. If you require additional breaks, your summit times will be greater.

If you are the fastest member of a group, it can be difficult to remember that the break begins, not ends, when the last person arrives. Make sure the stragglers also get five minutes to rest their legs and eat some food. If you are antsy to get going, volunteer to fill water bottles to take your attention off your watch.

What to Bring

One must balance safety, comfort, and weight when deciding what to bring on a hike. My basic rule is to carry sufficient gear to spend a night (albeit an unpleasant one) in the mountains. Most injuries occur late in the day, when you are tired and walking downhill. If your injury means you need assistance getting off the mountain, it will probably not arrive until the following morning. In other words, don't plan on being saved right away by one of the 200 others who will be on the same trail. This is a tall mountain in a remote wilderness, and the number of others on the trail is meaningless if you are alone or off the trail at the time of a serious accident.

Second, always remember you are carrying extra clothes and a first-aid kit for an emergency that could occur on the summit, not just an incident halfway up or down. Temperatures will be much cooler and winds stronger near the summit. Therefore, even if it's a warm and beautiful day, don't be tempted to stash your emergency gear halfway up the trail. And also don't get too upset with my recommendations when you descend from the summit having never worn more than shorts, a T-shirt, and maybe a windbreaker on the summit. I often wear none of the warm clothes I carry, but I never ascend to high elevation without them.

I have divided my recommendations on what to pack into four sections: footwear, the 10 essentials, additional gear for a dayhike, and additional gear for a backpacking trip. (Backpackers will need to read through all lists.) A checklist of the items in each of the lists is provided on page 80.

FOOTWEAR

It is difficult to advise others on appropriate hiking footwear, as each person's feet (and ankles and knees) have different needs. The only consensus among the people I've hiked with is to wear a pair of comfortable, well broken-in, but not worn-out shoes on a long hike. These shoes could be full leather hiking boots, lightweight cloth and leather hiking boots, trail runners, or lightweight running shoes.

Full disclosure: I'm biased toward heavy hiking boots, which provide the ankle and foot support that I require. In lighter shoes, I end up with very sore feet. I also appreciate being able to walk through creeks or snow without getting wet feet. The downside is that I often get blisters, but I successfully combat them with multiple layers of sports tape, applied before I start walking. Some years back, I stopped trying to convince friends that such boots were the best solution, because they kept coming back from trips—even off-trail, talus-hopping, rocky Sierra expeditions—complaining that they wished they had worn running shoes. They disliked having to pick up a heavy boot every step of the way, they got bad blisters, and they ended up with sore feet.

The moral is that making sure you have the right pair of shoes to wear to the summit of Mt. Whitney is as important as making sure you're in shape for the hike. These should be shoes that you have worn on many practice hikes, so that you know their shortcomings (if any) and have a plan to combat problems likely to occur.

Here are a few footwear suggestions that should transcend the "lightweight" versus "lots of support" debate:

- Consider bringing more than one pair of footwear. Before my first hike up Mt. Whitney, a friend advised me to wear running shoes to Trail Camp and then switch into hiking boots for the upper portion of the trail. This meant I had to haul hiking boots up the first 6 miles. But the advantage was that I got to wear lightweight, shock-absorbent shoes for the lower, sandier stretches of trail, and hiking boots with good ankle support and a tough tread for the higher-elevation, rockier sections of trail.

- If you wear trail runners, don't choose a pair with a tall, hiking bootlike "platform." This elevates your foot above the ground and raises your foot's center of gravity. Since you do not have any ankle support, this increases your chances of twisting an ankle, but it has no advantages.
- Don't wear old running shoes with worn-out padding. You will take approximately 75,000 steps on this hike, which will make any foot sore in a worn-out shoe.
- Bring an extra pair of socks. If your feet start to feel beat up on the descent, switch to a clean pair of socks with not-yet-compressed padding to give your feet new life.
- Wear a pair of ankle-high gaiters to keep pebbles and sand out of your shoes. Keeping the inside of your shoes clean reduces the likelihood of blisters.

TEN ESSENTIALS

The oft-mentioned list of 10 essentials covers nearly everything you will need for a summer dayhike up the Mt. Whitney Trail. The official list is: map, compass, sunglasses and sunscreen, extra food and water, extra clothes, headlamp or flashlight, first-aid kit, fire starter, matches, and a knife. To elaborate:

1. **Map:** Simply put, it is dangerous to be in the mountains without a map. Although you're unlikely to get lost along the Mt. Whitney Trail, if you wander off the trail (as may happen in the dark) or mistakenly take the wrong trail junction (as do many people at the junction with the John Muir Trail, especially on the descent), you need to determine where you are and how to return to the trail. The *Mt. Whitney* map from Wilderness Press or Tom Harrison's *Mt. Whitney Zone* map are excellent choices. (While a GPS unit can provide the same information, remember it runs on batteries might stop working if dropped.)

2. **Compass:** The only time you are likely to use a compass is if you become disoriented and need to orient your map, identify some basic landmarks, and thereby determine the direction to

RADIATION AT HIGH ELEVATION

The "light" emitted from the sun includes visible light, heat, and ultraviolet (UV) rays. Of these, UV rays are the highest energy and therefore do the most damage to your body. UV radiation is further divided into UVA, UVB, and UVC. The atmosphere absorbs all of the UVC rays and most of the UVB rays, but little of the UVA; the rest hits you. And it doesn't just hit you from above: Snow reflects 80 percent of light rays (including UV rays), so wearing a hat is only the first layer of protection when traveling over snow, as the rays bounce back and hit you from below.

Meanwhile, thin cloud cover decreases UV radiation by only 10 percent, and shade (which is hard to find anyway on the Mt. Whitney Trail) decreases UV radiation by as little as 50 percent. (That's right, you should still be wearing a hat while sitting under a tree.) Moreover, UV radiation increases by about 4 percent for each 1000-foot increase in elevation: At 10,000 feet, it is 50 percent greater than at sea level, and at 14,000 feet, it is nearly 80 percent greater. The only way to avoid it is by covering yourself with clothes or sunscreen, and sunglasses.

the trail or which direction to follow the trail. (Note that many GPS units do not include a compass.)

3. **Sunglasses and sunscreen:** Sunscreen and sunglasses (and a wide-brimmed hat) are a must in the Alpine Zone. If you don't protect yourself from the sun, you could get more than a nasty burn. Repeated exposure can lead to skin cancer and cataracts. Your sunscreen and sunglasses should protect you against both UVA and UVB, your sunscreen should be at least SPF 30. To avoid chapped or split lips, I also suggest bringing lip balm that is at least SPF 15. Apply sunscreen at least twice during your long hike up Mt. Whitney.

4. **Food:** As discussed in the fuel section on page 44, you will burn thousands of calories on an ascent of Mt. Whitney, and it is unlikely you will consume as many calories as you will expend on your walk. Dayhikers should carry enough food to be able to eat a 200- to 500-calorie snack every two hours and a larger lunch on the summit. In addition, bring 50 percent extra food in case something goes wrong or you underestimated your

appetite. (Even experienced hikers find their appetite is unpredictable from day to day, especially at high elevation). Bring a variety of different foods and foods you expect to find palatable when you are exhausted and at high altitude, where many people find it difficult to eat.

My snacks tend to consist of energy bars, granola bars, nuts, dried fruit, cookies, and jerky with a slightly larger snack I call "lunch" that includes bread and toppings that I reserve for the summit. Easily digestible foods, like Gu, provide your body with a rapidly accessible supply of energy and are also generally more appetizing when you are exhausted. I also recommend mixing electrolyte mix into at least some of your water. Full-strength Gatorade or Hydralyte (my favorite) are too strong for me. Sometimes, in a separate bottle I mix a liter at half strength and drink it slowly throughout the day. Likewise, it is a good idea to eat salty foods.

HINT: Make sure you consume calories regularly, rather than pushing yourself after you begin to feel hungry; it can take your body a long time to regain its energy if you continue upward after you have depleted your muscle's energy stores.

5. **Water:** As described on page 42, staying hydrated is incredibly important in reducing the likelihood you will suffer from a headache, muscle cramps, or unnecessary fatigue. Hydration also lowers your susceptibility to altitude sickness. Also remember that your body needs you to balance water consumption with food intake—otherwise your electrolyte levels will decrease.

    On this hike, 5 to 9 quarts of water a day should be adequate for most people. A rule of thumb among mountaineers is if your urine is a light yellow color, you are well-hydrated. This is very useful on an expedition up a remote, snow-covered mountain. Unfortunately, when you (especially if you are a woman) are trying to sneak behind a small boulder on the Mt. Whitney Trail and quickly pee into the gray gravel underfoot, you don't necessarily get a good look at your urine. Instead, at each break, check your water supply and make sure it is disappearing at the rate of a quart every 2 to 3 miles.

    It is also important to pack a hydration system or water bottle that has a capacity of at least a gallon. For the first 6 miles, you will cross a stream every few miles, but there is no water from the spring a few hundred feet above Trail Camp to the summit. This means that for 8.8 miles of the hike, when you are at the highest elevations, you cannot refill your water bottles. Many people leave the summit with empty water bottles—a bad idea. I leave the final water source carrying one gallon of water.

In addition to carrying enough water up the mountain, you actually need to drink it. During your training and acclimation hikes, determine a system that works for you. I highly recommend a bladder-and-tube hydration system like the CamelBak. I nearly doubled my water consumption when I switched to this system, because I drank a few sips every five minutes, whereas I'd previously procrastinated on taking out my water bottle until I was really thirsty—once every half hour at best. If it's a cool day and you're not inclined to drink much, you may want to set a watch alarm to beep every five or 10 minutes to remind yourself to take a few sips.

Lastly, if you plan to treat or filter your water, pack the appropriate device. See page 42 for a description of options.

HINT: Before you head up Mt. Whitney, determine a water-carrying and consuming method that works for you. For instance, a bladder-and-tube hydration system lets you drink as you are walking, letting you slowly and steadily consume water throughout your hike. Alternatively, carrying a water bottle lets you efficiently gulp large quantities of water, but you need to be disciplined to stop frequently to drink.

6. **Extra clothes:** You should carry sufficient clothes to spend a night out on the trail—up to an elevation of 14,505 feet. If you get lost or injure yourself late in the day, a rescue is unlikely until morning. At minimum, bring thermal tops and bottoms, a fleece hat, and a waterproof, wind-resistant jacket. Adding a fleece top and a pair of polypropylene gloves will greatly increase your comfort if a problem occurs, yet weigh less than a pound. If you are hiking early or late in the season, when you may encounter snow, throw in an extra pair of socks, as you may end up with wet feet. (If you don't own clothing made from fancy outdoor fabrics, it doesn't mean you'll be unsafe. Make sure you bring a warm, non-cotton top and a pair of non-cotton pants.)

7. **Headlamp or flashlight:** Nearly everyone walks part of this trail in the dark and will therefore need a light source. A headlamp is preferable, since it lets you have both hands free. My favorites are light-emitting diode (LED) headlamps,

HINT: When walking downhill in the dark, I sometimes hold my headlamp at waist level, as I make more shadows that highlight irregularities in the trail when lighting the path at this angle.

which weigh only a few ounces and run on a triplet of AAA batteries for at least 50 hours—the light gets dimmer with time but never quite gives out. In addition, the dimmer, diffuse light from the LEDs is better for walking than the brighter, more directed light from incandescent bulbs: Your pupils remain sufficiently dilated to see the edge of the trail, and irregularities in the trail surface stand out better. Indeed, I prefer half-used batteries for night walks.

8. **First-aid kit:** Your first-aid kit will most likely be used to prevent and treat blisters, limit an altitude-induced headache, and dull the pain from sore knees. If you sustain a serious injury, it also needs to keep you comfortable and medically stabilized, in case you need to wait to be evacuated.

A basic first-aid kit for a dayhike or short backpacking trip should contain:

- **Sports tape:** This essential first-aid component can be used to prevent or treat blisters, to tape anything in place, and to provide compression. An ideal anti-blister tape stays in place for many days, but isn't too thick. I am very fond of simple, thin, cheap sports tape. If I use long pieces, it stays put and doesn't add bulk to my feet. However, many people complain that cheap sports tape rubs off very easily, especially if you have sweaty feet. Some recommend using duct tape, which I dislike, because duct tape makes a permanent sticky mess of socks. Other suggestions for thicker, very sticky tapes include Leukoplast (only available in Europe/Australia/New Zealand, but adored by all hikers from those regions).

- **Anti-inflammatory pain medication:** For mild pain relief and to relieve swelling following an injury, ibuprofen, aspirin, and naproxen are all available over the counter. Acetaminophen is not an anti-inflammatory drug, but it is a very effective painkiller. Of these, ibuprofen and acetaminophen are easier on your stomach. If you take any of these, make sure you are well hydrated (to avoid kidney damage) and follow the indications on the product or the advice of your physician.

- **Moleskin, blister bandages, or pads:** Examples of blister bandages include Spenco 2nd Skin Blister Pads and Band-Aid Blister Block Cushions. Blister pads are expensive but highly recommended by people with persistent blister problems: They are gel pads that keep out dirt and germs, while providing cushioning, so your blister won't bother you for the rest of your hike.

- **Elastic bandage:** With an elastic bandage, you may be able to make slow progress down the trail with a strained or sprained ankle or knee. You can also use sports tape for this purpose.
- **Sterile gauze or adhesive pads:** These are handy to halt bleeding of a wound. There are many inexpensive brands of adhesive pads to cover wounds. The more expensive Tegaderm adhesive pads are permeable to water, vapor, and oxygen, but they provide a barrier to microorganisms, making them ideal if you can't reach a doctor within a few hours. Sanitary pads can also be used for this purpose, although they won't breathe.
- **Bandages:** Carry a variety of sizes, including butterfly closures. Band-Aids are great for any small cuts, while Steri-Strips can effectively close a larger wound to reduce bleeding.
- **Antibiotic ointment:** Apply antibiotic ointment (triple-action formulas are best) to a wound before dressing it.
- **Antiseptic wipes:** Use these to clean a wound before applying dressing.
- **Antihistamine:** Carry an over-the-counter antihistamine in case you have an allergic reaction or allergies. If you are severely allergic to something, you may need to carry something prescription strength, like an EpiPen.
- **Whistle and signal mirror:** Use these to attract attention to yourself if you are alone when injured.
- **Tweezers:** Use these to remove splinters.
- **Safety pin:** These are useful for fashioning clothing into slings or large bandages. Large, sturdy ones are handy for small repairs, from broken zippers to backpack straps. Zip ties also work well for fixing broken backpacks.
- **Sterile, non-latex gloves:** Wear these if you are treating an open wound on another person.
- **Small first-aid book:** Pamphlet-sized books are available at most outdoor stores.

Other items you may choose to carry in your first-aid kit include:

- Wire splint
- Chemical hand-warmer packets

- Prescription pain medication
- Anti-diarrhea drug, such as loperamide
- Knee brace

9. **Fire starter and matches:** These are important safety items to carry, always living in my backpack. Along the Mt. Whitney Trail, they should be used only in an emergency, and then only to create a smoke signal to help rescuers pinpoint your location. It is against the Forest Service regulations to build a fire along the entire length of the Mt. Whitney Trail. Moreover, above Mirror Lake, there is little to nothing to burn—and tugging away at the very slow-growing shrubs and trees would do enormous environmental damage. Be sure to carry sufficient clothing to survive a night at any elevation along the trail.

10. **Knife:** A small pocket knife, especially one with a pair of scissors, is important for cutting first-aid supplies—and probably for preparing your lunch.

DAYHIKE GEAR

In addition to the 10 essentials, dayhikers should carry the following:

- **Daypack:** Any small backpack will work. Some daypacks that are covered with gadgets and many small pockets can weigh 4 or more pounds, but they aren't necessary for this hike. Pick a simple one. Some people prefer a hip pack, but make sure you bring one that can accommodate a gallon of water.
- **Water-treatment method:** See page 42 for options.
- **Space blanket:** A space blanket costs less than $5, weighs about 3 ounces, and can help you retain body heat. Bring one to reduce the possibility of hypothermia if you spend an unplanned night on the mountain. I consider this as important as the 10 essentials.
- **Wag Bag:** You will receive one of these human-waste disposal kits free when you pick up your wilderness permit. Although they include a small amount of toilet paper, you may want to bring additional supplies. See page 78 for more information.

Optional items include:

- **Trekking poles:** Increasing numbers of hikers carry trekking poles. Their many advantages include taking weight off your knees, transferring some of the "work" to your arms, and providing extra balance, thereby minimizing your risk of falling.

- **Camera:** A camera is hardly optional for most people setting out for Mt. Whitney, but it's not required for your safety.
- **Altimeter:** You might find that the climb passes more quickly (or more slowly!) if you can watch yourself making continual progress.
- **Insect repellent:** During June and early July, the section of the trail between Lone Pine Lake and Mirror Lake may be home to swarming mosquitoes. If you march steadily through this area without any breaks, they shouldn't be too bothersome.

OVERNIGHT GEAR

In addition to the 10 essentials and the dayhike gear, backpackers should carry the items in this section. I provide few details on the different sorts of backpacks, tents, sleeping bags, and stoves—many

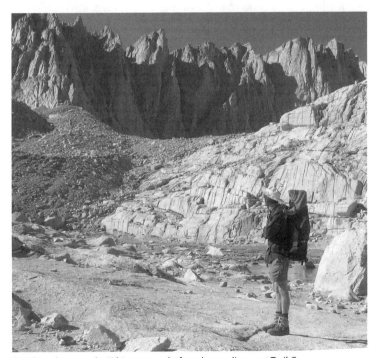

One last glance to the Whitney crest before descending past Trail Camp

books are written on these subjects and much information is available on the web and at outdoor stores if you are planning to buy new gear for this excursion.

- **Overnight backpack:** Either an internal or external frame backpack works well.
- **Additional clothes:** In addition to the clothes in the 10 essentials list, make sure you have a warm fleece jacket and a pair of wind pants. During June or September, you might choose to bring a down vest or jacket to make your evening at 12,000 feet more pleasant.

HUMAN WASTE ON THE MT. WHITNEY TRAIL

Until the summer of 2007, composting outhouses existed at Outpost Camp and Trail Camp. Unfortunately, the cool, dry climate in the mountains is not conducive to rapid decomposition, and the substantial use each season rapidly overwhelmed the toilets. Barrels of human waste had to be taken out by helicopter. Inyo National Forest decided this was not a sustainable solution and began phasing in a "pack out your waste" campaign in 2006.

In 2007, the toilets were removed and their previous locations so well restored it is difficult to pinpoint where they once stood. (The toilet that once stood at the summit of Mt. Whitney saw a similar end in 2006 for this reason.) When you pick up your permit, you'll be given a Wag Bag to pack out human waste. The kits consist of two concentric bags: The inner bag has an absorptive powder that both deodorizes and helps decay solid waste, and the outer bag zips closed for easy transport. They do a remarkable job of not reeking.

There are specially marked bins at Whitney Portal in which to deposit your used bags. A side benefit of removing the toilets is that backpackers are now less inclined to camp only at Outpost Camp and Trail Camp. There are plenty of other beautiful little sandy shelves between Mirror Lake and Trail Camp that are suddenly being used again. The only downside: It is very hard to find privacy along the trail to do your business.

- **Sleeping bag:** In summer, if you are a warm sleeper, a 30°F to 35°F bag should suffice, while cooler sleepers will prefer a 20°F bag.
- **Ground pad:** Either a closed-cell foam pad or an inflatable mattress works well. To save weight, I carry a short pad and place clothes and my empty backpack under my feet.
- **Tent, tarp, or bivy sack:** If the weather forecast is for clear skies, a tent isn't necessary—although it is a good windbreak and provides extra warmth. Also note that mosquitoes are not much of a problem at Trail Camp, but might be pesky at Outpost Camp. Despite what many detractors say, it is perfectly feasible to pitch a non-free-standing tent in the Sierra, even on slabs or shallow soil; you just have to be creative with string and rocks.
- **Stove and fuel:** Most choices will work, but note that fuel canisters do not work as well as white gas stoves at high elevation or in the cold.
- **Pot:** Any lightweight camping pot works well. One 2-liter pot works well for groups of one to three, while larger groups might choose to carry a second pot.
- **Bear canister:** Bear-resistant food canisters are required along the Mt. Whitney Trail. The Sierra Interagency Black Bear Group website (www.sierrawildbear.gov/foodstorage/ approvedcontainers.htm) lists the bear canisters approved for use in the Sierra Nevada. Of these, the Garcia canisters are the most widely available and can be rented from any Inyo National Forest ranger station, usually for $5 per trip (no reservations necessary). I use the lighter-weight Bearikade canister that can be bought or rented only from the manufacturer, Wild Ideas (805-693-0550 or www.wild-ideas.net/index2.html).
- **Additional food:** In addition to lunch and snacks, be sure to carry hearty breakfasts and dinners. I always start my dinner with a cup of instant soup. My body needs the salt and enjoys the warm liquid.
- **Eating utensils** and eating container
- **A simple toiletry kit:** This should include a toothbrush and toothpaste, personal medications, extra toilet paper, and tampons or sanitary pads, if applicable. Keep it simple, since toiletries need to be stored in your bear canister at night.

PACKING CHECKLIST

Note: Items in *italics* are optional.

	Dayhike	Overnight
☐ Daypack	●	●
☐ Overnight backpack		●
Route-Finding		
☐ Map (*or GPS*)	●	●
☐ Compass	●	●
Sun Protection		
☐ Sunglasses	●	●
☐ Sunscreen (SPF 30+)	●	●
☐ Lip balm (SPF 15+)	●	●
☐ Sunhat with ear protection	●	●
☐ Food	●	●
☐ Water bottles/hydration system	●	●
Clothes		
☐ Shoes	●	●
☐ Wool or synthetic socks	●	●
☐ Fleece or wool hat	●	●
☐ Thermal bottoms	●	●
☐ Thermal tops	●	●
☐ Fleece top		●
☐ Rain/wind jacket	●	●
☐ Wind pants		●
☐ Hiking shirt	●	●
☐ Hiking shorts or pants	●	●
☐ *Gaiters*	●	●
☐ *Extra socks*	●	●
☐ *Gloves*	●	●
First-Aid Kit		
☐ Sports tape	●	●
☐ Pain medication	●	●
☐ Moleskin/blister bandages	●	●

	Dayhike	Overnight
☐ Elastic bandage	•	•
☐ Sterile gauze and adhesive pads	•	•
☐ Miscellaneous bandages	•	•
☐ Antibiotic ointment	•	•
☐ Antiseptic wipes	•	•
☐ Antihistamine	•	•
☐ Whistle and signal mirror	•	•
☐ Tweezers	•	•
☐ Safety pin	•	•
☐ Sterile gloves	•	•
☐ First-aid book	•	•

Miscellaneous

	Dayhike	Overnight
☐ Headlamp	•	•
☐ Fire starter	•	•
☐ Matches	•	•
☐ Knife	•	•
☐ Water treatment	•	•
☐ Space blanket	•	•
☐ Wag bag and toilet paper	•	•
☐ *Trekking poles*	•	•
☐ *Camera*	•	•
☐ *Altimeter*	•	•
☐ *Insect repellent*	•	•
☐ Tent/shelter		•
☐ Sleeping bag		•
☐ Ground pad		•
☐ Stove		•
☐ Stove fuel		•
☐ Cooking pot		•
☐ Eating utensil		•
☐ Eating vessel		•
☐ Bear canister		•
☐ Toiletry kit		•

Getting There

The small town of Lone Pine is located at the eastern base of the Sierra, 13 linear miles east of the summit of Mt. Whitney. If you're coming from out of town to hike Mt. Whitney, Lone Pine or one of the campgrounds near the trailhead, Whitney Portal, will be your base. Lone Pine is located along Hwy. 395 in the Owens Valley in southeastern California; by car, it is approximately four hours north of Los Angeles, seven hours southeast of San Francisco, and five hours south of Reno, Nevada.

The following directions are written from the major airports. Please consult a map for additional information.

From Los Angeles International Airport in western Los Angeles: As you exit the airport, head east on Interstate 105. After 1.5 miles, exit and drive north on Interstate 405, toward Santa Monica. Continue for 29 miles to the junction between Interstate 5 and Hwy. 14. Drive north on Hwy. 14 for 118 miles to the Hwy. 395 junction near Ridgecrest. Continue north on Hwy. 395 for 65 miles to Lone Pine. Total distance: 214 miles.

From Ontario International Airport in eastern Los Angeles: Exit the airport onto Interstate 10, and head east, toward San Bernardino. After 2.5 miles, drive on Interstate 15, and continue for 30 miles to the Hwy. 395 junction. Take Hwy. 395 north for 164 miles to Lone Pine. Total distance: 197 miles.

From San Diego International Airport: From the airport, head south on Interstate 5, but turn north onto Hwy. 163 after 0.5 mile. After 10.5 miles, merge north onto Interstate 15 and continue north for 127 miles. Shortly before Hesperia, turn north on Hwy. 395 and follow it 164 miles to Lone Pine. Total distance: 302 miles.

From the San Francisco International Airport: Head south on Hwy. 101 for 7 miles and then turn east onto Hwy. 92, toward Hayward. After 14 miles, you reach Interstate 880 and head north for 3.5 miles. Now turn onto Interstate 238 south, which you follow for 3 miles until it merges with Interstate 580. Head east on Interstate 580, continuing for 29 miles, until you are east of Altamont Pass at the junction between Interstate 580 and Hwy. 205.

You then have the choice of heading north, via Yosemite National Park, or heading south down the Central Valley. Both routes require a similar amount of time from this junction.

If you head north, take Hwy. 205 for 13.5 miles to Interstate 5. Drive north on Interstate 5 for 2 miles, and then turn east onto Hwy. 120. After 6 miles, turn north onto Hwy. 99. Continue for 2 miles, and then continue east on Hwy. 120. Follow Hwy. 120 through Oakdale, the Sierra foothills, and through Yosemite National Park to Lee Vining, a distance of 155 miles. From Lee Vining (east of Yosemite), drive south on Hwy. 395 for 121 miles. The only words of warning: Hwy. 120 through Yosemite National Park is usually closed from late October until at least Memorial Day weekend, and you'll have to pay the National Park Service entrance fee to drive through Yosemite. Total distance: 357 miles.

If you choose to head south, continue an additional 17 miles on Interstate 580 to Interstate 5, follow Interstate 5 south for 167 miles, and then turn east onto Hwy. 46 and follow it for 25 miles to Hwy. 99. Head south on Hwy. 99 for 20 miles, taking you to Bakersfield. In Bakersfield, turn east onto Hwy. 58, and follow it for 58 miles across Tehachapi Pass to the Hwy. 14 junction. Head north on Hwy. 14 for 44 miles, and then merge with Hwy. 395, heading north for an additional 65 miles to Lone Pine. Total distance: 455 miles.

From Reno-Tahoe International Airport: Drive south on Hwy. 395 for 257 miles.

Once you reach Lone Pine, here are directions for getting to Whitney Portal: The Mt. Whitney Trail trailhead lies 13 miles west of Lone Pine (Hwy. 395 doubles as Lone Pine's Main Street). Turn west at the only stoplight in town onto Whitney Portal Road. The road winds through the Alabama Hills and eventually climbs steeply up to Whitney Portal. (See page 91 for a map of Whitney Portal.)

Lone Pine and Whitney Portal

Beginning around 1863, people began to inhabit Lone Pine to pro-vide supplies for the nearby mining towns; by the 1920s, Lone Pine became a hub for the film industry, especially for westerns. Since then, 300 films have been shot in the surrounding Alabama Hills. The declining popularity of westerns in the 1950s brought fewer film crews to Lone Pine, but even today, commercials and films are regularly shot in Owens Valley (where Lone Pine is located)—the desert foreground flanked by steep mountains is an undeniably dra-matic setting. (To learn more about Lone Pine's movie history, visit the Lone Pine Film Museum; see page 130 for details.)

Whitney Portal, the trailhead for Mt. Whitney, was established fol-lowing the construction of the Whitney Portal Road between 1933 and 1935. The private cabins near the Whitney Portal campground were erected beginning in 1934, and the Whitney Portal Store was built in 1935. The store, a mainstay of the Whitney experience that serves food off the grill and hosts a fantastic web message board (www.whitneyportalstore.com), has been run by its current own-ers, Doug and Earlene Thompson, since 1987. It is also packed with last-minute essentials you need for your hike, including snacks, ponchos, and maps. Many people doing the Mt. Whitney Trail as a three-day trip plan to return to Whitney Portal before 11 AM to get a plate of pancake. (Yes, that's "pancake," not "pancakes." It is so large, they'll give you your money back if you can finish it.) Also, grab a copy of the Thompson's book, *Mount Whitney: Mountain Lore from the Whitney Store* (Westwind Publishing Company, 2003) for more stories and tidbits about Whitney's history.

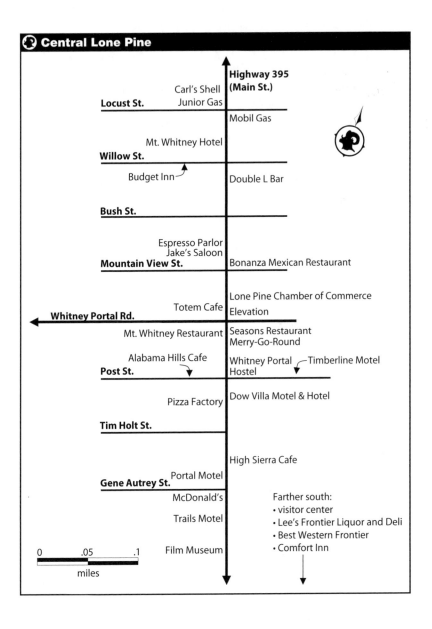

Central Lone Pine

Highway 395
(Main St.)

Carl's Shell
Junior Gas

Locust St.

Mobil Gas

Mt. Whitney Hotel

Willow St.

Budget Inn

Double L Bar

Bush St.

Espresso Parlor
Jake's Saloon

Mountain View St.

Bonanza Mexican Restaurant

Lone Pine Chamber of Commerce

Totem Cafe   Elevation

Whitney Portal Rd.

Mt. Whitney Restaurant   Seasons Restaurant
Merry-Go-Round

Alabama Hills Cafe

Post St.

Whitney Portal   Timberline Motel
Hostel

Pizza Factory   Dow Villa Motel & Hotel

Tim Holt St.

High Sierra Cafe

Portal Motel

Gene Autrey St.

McDonald's

Trails Motel

Farther south:
• visitor center
• Lee's Frontier Liquor and Deli
• Best Western Frontier
• Comfort Inn

Film Museum

0   .05   .1

miles

Lodging and Camping

Due to the popularity of the Owens Valley and Whitney region of the Sierra Nevada as tourist destinations, there are many nearby lodging and camping choices. Most of the independently owned motels in Lone Pine have similar prices. The newly opened and economical Whitney Portal Hostel is run by the Thompsons, the Whitney Portal Store owners. At the hostel are five public showers ($5) open 24 hours a day. Campgrounds exist on both public land and on land owned by the Los Angeles Department of Water and Power. Staying at the higher-elevation campgrounds is recommended during the summer: Temperatures are more pleasant, and camping up high will help your body acclimate. For additional information about lodging in Lone Pine, visit the Lone Pine Chamber of Commerce website at www.lonepinechamber.org.

LONE PINE HOTELS AND MOTELS

Best Western Frontier
1008 S. Main Street
760-876-5571 or 1-800-528-1234

Budget Inn & Hotel
138 W. Willow Street
760-876-5655 or 1-877-283-4381

Comfort Inn
1920 S. Main Street
760-876-8700 or 1-800-800-6468

Dow Villa Motel & Hotel
310 S. Main Street
760-876-5521 or 1-800-824-9317

Mt. Whitney Motel
305 N. Main Street
760-876-4207 or 1-800-845-2362

Portal Motel
425 S. Main Street
760-876-5930 or 1-800-531-7054

Timberline Motel
215 E. Post Street
760-876-4555 or 1-800-862-7020

Trails Motel
633 S. Main Street
760-876-5555

Whitney Portal Hostel
238 S. Main Street
760-876-0030

RV FACILITIES

Boulder Creek RV Resort
2550 S. Main Street (Hwy. 395, 4 miles south of Lone Pine)
760-876-4243 or 1-800-648-8965

CAMPING

Note: None of these camping options offer RV hookups.

Inyo National Forest: For campgrounds in this section that accept reservations, you can reserve online at www.fs.fed.us/r5/inyo/recreation/campgrounds.shtml.

Whitney Trailhead
Located adjacent to the Whitney Portal parking area, this campground has 10 first-come, first-served walk-in sites. One night stay only. *Price:* $8 per site. *Amenities:* water, pit toilets.

Whitney Portal and Whitney Portal Group
Located 1 mile east of Whitney Portal, at the Meysan Lakes Trailhead on the Whitney Portal Road, this campsite has 43 sites and three group sites, all of which are available by reservation. Camping at Whitney Portal the night before your hike will help your body acclimate, so this is a good spot to choose if you plan to dayhike the mountain. *Price:* $16 per traditional campsite and $45 per group site. *Amenities:* water, flush toilets.

Lone Pine and Lone Pine Group
Located off Whitney Portal Road: From Lone Pine, drive 6.5 miles west on the Whitney Portal Road and look for the campground on the south side of the road. There are 43 campsites and one group site here, all of which are available by reservation. *Price:* $14 per traditional site and $45 per group site. *Amenities:* water, pit toilets.

Bureau of Land Management:

Tuttle Creek
Located off Horseshoe Meadows Road: From Lone Pine, drive 3.5 miles west on the Whitney Portal Road, and turn left (south) to drive 1.5 miles on the Horseshoe Meadows Road. From there, follow signs to the campground. Tuttle Creek has 85 first-come, first-served campsites. *Price:* $5 per site. *Amenities:* pit toilets, but no potable water.

Los Angeles Department of Water and Power:

Portagee Joe
Located off Whitney Portal Road: From Lone Pine, drive less than 1 mile west on the Whitney Portal Road, and turn left (south) to drive 0.1 mile on Tuttle Creek Road. This campground has 15 sites, which you can reserve by calling 760-873-5577. *Price:* $10 per site. *Amenities:* water, pit toilets.

Diaz Lake County Park
Located on the west side of Hwy. 395, 2 miles south of Lone Pine, this campground has 200 sites, which you can reserve by calling 760-876-5656. *Price:* $14 per site. *Amenities:* water, flush toilets.

Restaurants

Lone Pine has plenty of restaurants to choose between, from fast food to pricier, but very tasty steak houses. A selection of menu items are provided. Note that only summer hours are listed.

Whitney Portal Store
Located at Whitney Portal
760-876-0030
Hours: June and September, 8 AM to 8 PM; July and August, 7 AM to 9 PM. *Menu:* breakfast, burgers, sandwiches, and more off the grill

Alabama Hills Cafe and Bakery
111 W. Post Street
760-876-4675
Hours: Wednesday through Monday, 5:30 AM to 2 PM; closed Tuesday. *Menu:* freshly baked bread, breakfast, burgers, sandwiches, pasta, and steak

Bonanza Mexican Restaurant
104 N. Main Street
760-876-4768
Hours: Saturday through Sunday, 8 AM to 8 PM; Monday through Friday, 11 AM to 8 PM. *Menu:* full selection of Mexican food

Carl's Junior
403 N. Main Street
760-876-1035
Hours: Friday, 6:30 AM to 11 PM; Saturday through Thursday, 6:30 AM to 10 PM. *Menu:* burgers and other fast food

Espresso Parlor
123 N. Main Street
760-876-9110
Hours: Daily, 6 AM to 7 PM. *Menu:* coffee, espresso drinks, and smoothies

High Sierra Cafe
446 S. Main Street
760-876-5796
Hours: 24 hours a day. *Menu:* Full selection of classic diner food, including breakfast, sandwiches, and dinner; the only option for a 3 AM breakfast out before hitting the trail

Lee's Frontier Liquor and Deli
1900 S. Main Street (next to the Chevron)
760-876-5844
Hours: Daily, 4 AM to 8 PM. *Menu:* deli sandwiches, soup, and fried chicken

McDonald's
601 S. Main Street
760-876-4355 or 760-876-4366
Hours: Daily, 5 AM to 9 PM. *Menu:* burgers and other fast food

Merry-Go-Round
212 S. Main Street
760-876-4115
Hours: Daily, 5 PM to 10 PM. *Menu:* steaks and seafood

Mt. Whitney Restaurant
227 S. Main Street
760-876-5751
Hours: Daily, 6:30 AM to 9 PM. *Menu:* Breakfast, lunch, and dinner; specializes in a diverse selection of burgers, including venison, buffalo, and ostrich

Pizza Factory
301 S. Main Street
760-876-4707
Hours: Friday and Saturday, 11 AM to 10 PM; Sunday through Thursday, 11 AM to 9 PM. *Menu:* Pizza and salad

Seasons Restaurant
206 S. Main Street
760-876-8927
Hours: Daily, 5 PM to 10 PM. *Menu:* steak and seafood

Totem Cafe
131 S. Main Street
760-876-1120
Hours: Daily, 7 AM to 9 PM. *Menu:* breakfast, sandwiches, burgers, steak, and seafood

Outdoor Equipment Shops

Elevation, Sierra Adventure Essentials
125 N. Main Street
760-876-4560
Note: This is Lone Pine's only well-outfitted mountaineering shop, with equipment rentals available, even after hours (the owner's number is on the store door).

Gardner's Home and Sporting Center
(True Value Hardware)
104 S. Main Street
760-876-4208

High Sierra Outfitters
130 S. Main Street
760-876-9994

Lone Pine Sporting Goods
220 S. Main Street
760-876-5365

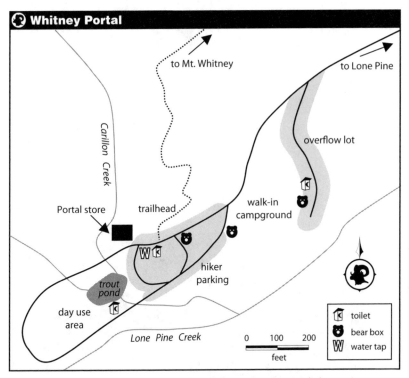

The layout of Whitney Portal is really quite straightforward—when it is light out. As you're trying to get organized to start hiking at 2 AM, it helps to know in advance where to find bear boxes, the water tap, toilets, and the trailhead.

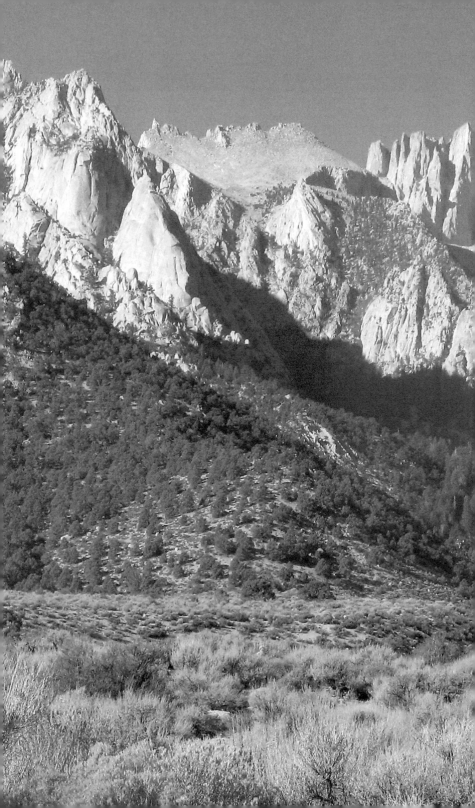

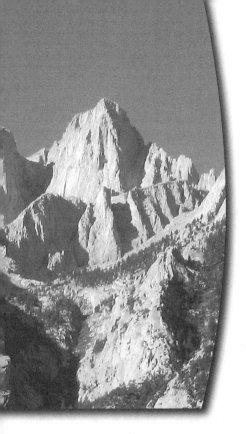

4
Hiking
Mt. Whitney

How Long It Takes

The amount of time you require to reach the summit is determined by your pace and the time you spend taking breaks. The formula is different for each person, and the optimal solution for you can only be determined through practice. When you are on training hikes, try different walking paces on different days, to learn how your lungs and legs feel under different conditions. Over time, you will discover a pace that feels "right."

There are two tricks to converting that knowledge into a successful hike up Mt. Whitney. First, take enough training hikes so that you know exactly how your lungs and legs feel when your pace is good, rather than how fast you were going on a given day. After all, the actual distance covered and elevation gained per time can be wildly different on different trails, but you'll have the same pairs of legs and lungs. Second, on a very long hike, such as this one, force yourself to go about 80 percent of your good pace, because you have a long way to go. I have hiked with many very fit, gung ho hikers who sped past me during the first hours of the walk but ran out of reserves long before the top and were unable to summit.

Opposite and above: Thor Peak and the Whitney crest, including Crooks Peak, Keeler Needle, and Mt. Whitney, from the Whitney Portal Road

DAYHIKE TIMING

The hike up the Mt. Whitney Trail to the summit of 14,505-foot Mt. Whitney is approximately 10.5 miles, with nearly 6500 feet of altitude gain. First-time dayhikers should expect the ascent to take between nine and 11 hours, especially because you are at high elevation. A quite fast time to the summit is between five and six hours.

Most people will find the descent faster, likely taking you between half as long to two-thirds as long. (The fastest round-trip time on the Whitney Trail is purported to be less than four hours.)

To determine when to leave, work backward from the latest acceptable return time—plan to be back at Whitney Portal an hour before dark. Going uphill in the dark isn't a problem, but at the end of a long day, it is simply too easy to trip walking downhill in the dark. (It is also more difficult to illuminate the trail while walking downhill.) In addition, if an accident does occur, you don't want it to be in the dark, when help will probably not arrive until the following morning.

The math to determine your trip time is as follows:

- Plan to take between nine and 11 hours to ascend. If this is your first time on such a long hike, it is, of course, difficult to estimate exactly how long it will take you. Based on conversations with a variety of first-timers, I've determined that most people climbing the mountain for the first time take nine hours, and about a quarter of hikers need at least 11 hours. (These estimates include 10 minutes of breaks for each hour. If you anticipate taking longer breaks on your ascent, give yourself extra time.)

SUGGESTED START TIMES FOR DAYHIKE

Month	7-hour Ascent (13-hour round trip)	9-hour Ascent (16-hour round trip)	11-hour Ascent (19-hour round trip)
June and July	6:45 AM	3:45 AM	12:45 AM
August	6:15 AM	3:15 AM	12:15 AM
September	5:30 AM	2:30 AM	11:30 PM

- Give yourself an hour on the summit.
- Plan to take between five and seven hours to descend.
- Plan to return an hour before dark. In June and July, it gets dark around 8:45 PM, in August it gets dark around 8:15 PM, and by mid-September, it is dark at 7:30 PM.

When planning your start time, be conservative. I recommend leaving no later than 6 AM, even if you expect to ascend quickly. The calculations described here do not take into account thunderstorm activity, which would mean you'd need to be off the summit by noon (thus requiring an earlier departure time). If you leave too early, the worst that happens is that you get to take a longer summit break or get back to Lone Pine for an earlier dinner. See the hike timetable on page 100 for more details.

BACKPACK TIMING

If you will be backpacking, your first day will be shorter in distance, elevation gain, and time, than if you plan to do Whitney in a day, but it is nonetheless a tough hike. The distance to either Outpost Camp (3.8 miles) or Trail Camp (6.15 miles) is unlikely to be the limiting factor. Instead, it is the relentless elevation gain: The trail goes straight up, and you gain approximately 2000 feet if you stay at Outpost Camp, and 3700 feet if you stay at Trail Camp. An average hiker will require four hours to reach Outpost Camp and nearly seven hours to reach Trail Camp. Between the trailhead and Mirror Lake (a 4.3-mile stretch), the trail is very hot midday, so it is best to start hiking by 8 AM and get the early miles under your belt before lunch. Arriving at your campsite early gives you time to relax and enjoy your surroundings.

How Long It Takes

Your choice of campsite (see next section) will determine the length of your approach hike as well as the time required to summit Mt. Whitney the next day. A rule of thumb is that it takes an hour to backpack 2 miles on flat ground, and you add an additional hour for each thousand feet of elevation gain. In effect, to reach Trail Camp, it takes:

6.15 miles ÷ 2 = 3.05 hours
3700 feet ÷ 1000 = 3.7 hours
Total one-way time = 6.75 hours

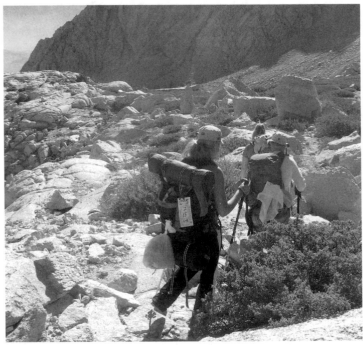

Descending toward Trailside Meadow after a successful climb

This time takes into account about 10 minutes of breaks per hour, but not lengthy lunches. Using this formula, the amount of time required to reach each of the suggested campsites is included in the table that follows. Excepting those wishing to bivy on or near the summit, there is plenty of daylight to reach these campsites, although I still recommend leaving by 8 AM to avoid ascending the lower stretches of the trail in the heat of the day. Once you reach camp, expect to spend two hours setting up camp, cooking, and eating dinner. Before retiring for the night, make sure you have an agreed upon wake-up time. Organize your summit pack, fill your water bottles, and pre-pack your lunch (and then store it inside your bear canister). Mornings are chilly at high elevation, and it is easy to forget something when it is dark and you are half asleep, so do as many of these tasks as possible the day before.

Although your summit day does not require as much of a pre-dawn start as it does for those dayhiking from Whitney Portal, you should still set out from Trail Camp between 6 AM and 7 AM and Outpost Camp between 4:30 AM and 6 AM—and perhaps an hour earlier if you want to take your time or need to return to Whitney Portal in the afternoon. The table on page 100 indicates how long you will likely require to summit. Remember to budget an extra hour to pack up camp once you have completed the summit, and also keep in mind that it will take you about half to two-thirds as long to descend as it did to ascend. Plan to be back at the trailhead an hour before dark.

Where to Camp

Along the Mt. Whitney Trail, backpackers have a limited selection of campsites, as there is relatively little flat real estate in the vicinity of water (see table on page 98). The largest sites are at Outpost Camp (at 10,365 feet) and Trail Camp (at 12,040 feet), and these are obviously well used, especially the ones at Trail Camp, where close to 50 people camp each night, all summer long. Fortunately, the underlying substrate is sandy, so these sites are not dusty like heavily used camps at lower elevations. In past years, nearly everyone stayed at Outpost Camp and Trail Camp to take advantage of the solar toilets. Now that these have been removed, people have begun to drift more toward the smaller sites.

A few small sites (at 10,860 feet) exist beneath foxtail pines on the slope above Mirror Lake, although the closest water is at least a 10-minute walk back down the trail to Mirror Lake. (Camping is prohibited along the banks of Mirror Lake.) Between Trailside Meadow (camping prohibited) and Trail Camp, there are scattered sites (between 11,500 and 11,900 feet) in sandy patches between granite slabs, mostly less than a five-minute walk from water. If you wish to camp farther from the trail, there are sites near the shores of Consultation Lake (11,680 feet) or south of Trail Camp.

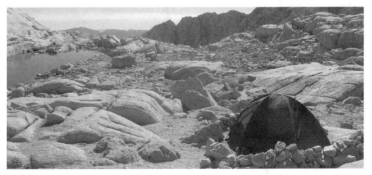

Trail Camp

Here are some considerations to make in deciding the best site for you:

- **Regulations:** Regulations detailed on your wilderness permit indicate you should camp 100 feet from the trail or water sources, and you should never camp on vegetation, including meadows. The fragile subalpine and alpine meadows can take years to recover from disturbance, so please take the ecology into account if you wander off the trail in search of a campsite. Camp only in sandy flats and previously used sites.

CAMPSITE LOCATIONS

Description	Distance from Whitney Portal (miles)
Lone Pine Lake: Sites beneath scattered lodgepole pine cover, especially on the ridge north of Lone Pine Lake	2.85
Outpost Camp: Large camping area beneath foxtail pines to the southwest of the creek crossing	3.8
Medium-sized site beneath foxtail pines; lovely site, but far from water	4.5
Small, sandy sites among slabs on open knob above Trailside Meadow	5.2
Many small, sandy sites among slabs along the trail a short distance before Trail Camp	5.8
Trail Camp: Many sites in sandy flats among slabs, on both sides of trail; additional, more isolated sites if you continue south from Trail Camp	6.15
Several small, very exposed, sandy, bivy sites among talus in the vicinity of the John Muir Trail junction; some below the Mt. Whitney Trail and others just below the Sierra Crest	8.5
Mt. Whitney summit: Various bivy sites on the summit plateau	10.5

- **Elevation:** If you camp higher, you put yourself at greater risk for altitude sickness, but you also will have a more leisurely summit day. Few people coming from low elevation sleep well at 12,000 feet, but the advantages of an alpine perch may outweigh the headache and lack of appetite the night before. Nonetheless, if you have never camped above 10,000 feet, and have not spent the previous day (or days) doing an acclimation hike, I recommend camping at Outpost Camp: You will probably sleep better and will therefore enjoy your hike to the summit.

Time from Whitney Portal (hours)	Time to Summit (hours)	Elevation (feet)	Approximate UTM Coordinates (NAD 27)
3:00	7:00	10,030	11S 388198E 4048277N
4:00	6:30	10,365	11S 387453E 4047897N
4:45	6:00	10,860	11S 387145E 4047628N
5:45	5:15	11,450	11S 386656E 4047421N
6:30	4:45	11,900	11S 386025E 4047057N
6:45	4:30	12,040	11S 385618E 4046947N
9:30	1:45	13,450	11S 384406E 4046780N
11:45	NA	14,505	11S 384474E 4048700N

The bivy sites near the John Muir Trail junction (13,450 feet) or on the summit of Mt. Whitney offer the most spectacular alpine views, but they are also cold, windy, and high enough that you'll be guaranteed to feel the elevation.

- **On trail or off trail:** There are advantages and disadvantages to camping on and off the trail. If you camp at the designated sites, you won't have to detour from the trail to search for a flat spot of sand. On the other hand, you'll have more privacy if you do take the time to find a site off trail.
- **Distance from summit:** Your summit day will be shorter if you select a higher campsite. However, do not force yourself to camp high if you are concerned that you will spend the night feeling sick due to the altitude—this will decrease you chances of summiting the next day.
- **Crowds:** The large number of tent sites at Outpost Camp and Trail Camp mean that you will have many neighbors at these locations. However, they are picturesque sites with very easy access to water and plenty of flat campsites.

HIKE TIMETABLE AND ITINERARY

Location	GPS (UTM) Coordinates (NAD 27)	Elevation (feet)
Whitney Portal Parking Lot	11S 389118E 4049568N	8330
North Fork of Lone Pine Creek	11S 388673E 4049563N	8720
Lone Pine Lake Junction	11S 388198E 4048277N	10,030
Outpost Camp	11S 387453E 4047897N	10,365
Mirror Lake	11S 387166E 4047791N	10,670
Trailside Meadow	11S 386611E 4047350N	11,420
Trail Camp	11S 385618E 4046947N	12,040
Trail Crest	11S 384523E 4046537N	13,635
"End of Pinnacles"	11S 384520E 4048013N	13,910
Mt. Whitney Summit	11S 384474E 4048700N	14,505

Figures in parentheses indicate cumulative information

The Hike Itself

The table below divides the hike up the Mt. Whitney Trail into nine sections, and includes necessary statistics for each part—distance, elevation gain, estimated timing, and UTM coordinates. The suggested time itinerary is provided for seven- nine-, and 11-hour ascents. The amount of time needed takes into account distance, elevation gain, and altitude (it assumes you will go more slowly the higher you get). While rest breaks are not explicitly indicated, this time table allows for 10 minutes of rest breaks per hour. In each case, the point-to-point and cumulative (in parentheses) information is provided. The elevation gain numbers include the extra ups and downs of the trail itself, so don't be confused when you see that the total climb is greater than the 6175-foot elevation difference between Whitney Portal and the summit of Mt. Whitney.

Distance (miles)	Elevation Gain (feet)	Timing for 11-hour Ascent	Timing for 9-hour Ascent	Timing for 7-hour Ascent
0.9 (0.9)	390 (390)	0:35 (0:35)	0:30 (0:30)	0:25 (0:25)
1.9 (2.8)	1310 (1700)	1:45 (2:20)	1:30 (2:00)	1:05 (1:30)
1.0 (3.8)	345 (2045)	0:40 (3:00)	0:30 (2:30)	0:25 (1:55)
0.5 (4.3)	305 (2350)	0:30 (3:30)	0:20 (2:50)	0:15 (2:10)
0.8 (5.1)	750 (3100)	1:00 (4:30)	0:50 (3:40)	0:40 (2:50)
1.0 (6.1)	620 (3720)	1:00 (5:30)	0:50 (4:30)	0:40 (3:30)
2.2 (8.3)	1595 (5315)	3:00 (8:30)	2:30 (7:00)	2:00 (5:30)
1.2 (9.5)	535 (5850)	1:15 (9:45)	1:00 (8:00)	0:45 (6:15)
1.0 (10.5)	600 (6450)	1:15 (11:00)	1:00 (9:00)	0:45 (7:00)

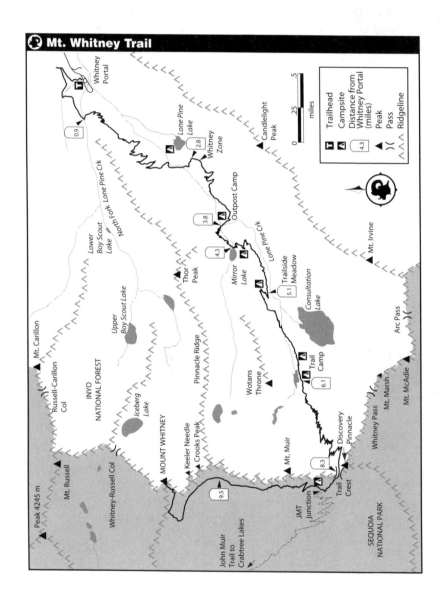

Mt. Whitney Trail

Whitney Portal

0.9

Lone Pine Lake

2.8

Whitney Zone

Candlelight Peak

miles

0   .25   .5

Trailhead

Campsite

Distance from Whitney Portal (miles)

4.3

Peak

Pass

Ridgeline

North Fork Lone Pine Crk

Lower Boy Scout Lake

Outpost Camp

3.8

Lone Pine Crk

Mt. Irvine

Thor Peak

4.3

Mirror Lake

Trailside Meadow

5.1

Consultation Lake

Upper Boy Scout Lake

Mt. Carillon

Russell-Carillon Col

INYO

NATIONAL FOREST

Iceberg Lake

Pinnacle Ridge

Wotans Throne

Trail Camp

6.1

Arc Pass

Mt. Russell

Whitney-Russell Col

MOUNT WHITNEY

Keeler Needle

Crooks Peak

Mt. Muir

Discovery Pinnacle

Whitney Pass

Mt. Marsh

Mt. McAdie

Mt. Mallory

Peak 4245 m

8.3

Trail Crest

9.5

JMT junction

John Muir Trail to Crabtree Lakes

SEQUOIA NATIONAL PARK

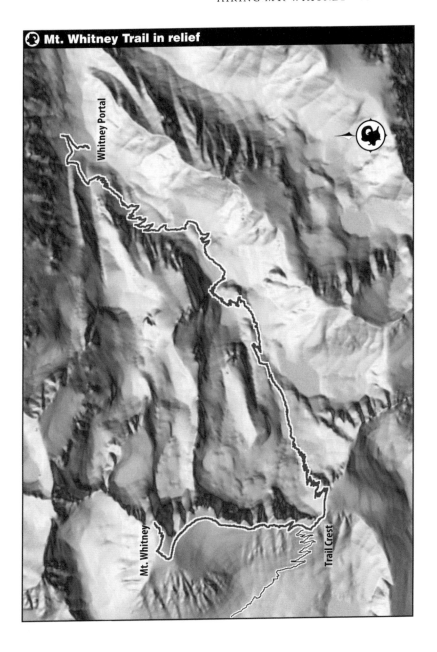

Mt. Whitney Trail in relief

Whitney Portal

Mt. Whitney

Trail Crest

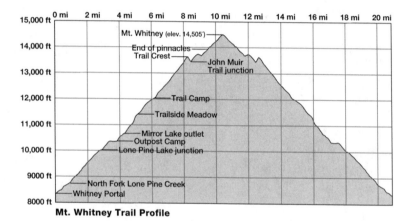

Mt. Whitney Trail Profile

**SECTION
1**

Parking Lot to the North Fork of Lone Pine Creek

Distance. . . . . 0.9 mile

Leaving the parking lot, head north for the sign pointing to the trailhead; you will pass large information plaques and a handy scale to weigh your pack. The trail begins by heading north, with a couple of quick switchbacks. After crossing a small creek, you emerge onto a dry, sandy slope. After about 0.3 mile, you complete an east-trending switchback, and begin a

HINT: Take your time getting started: Slow and steady is the mantra for success on this hike. Give your legs at least 15 minutes to warm up before speeding up to full pace—your leg muscles will thank you later.

long, westward traverse along the south side of the canyon. Gaining little elevation, you cross this open slope, which is dotted with drought-tolerant shrubs and sports an understory of colorful flowers in spring and early summer. Along the way, you cross several

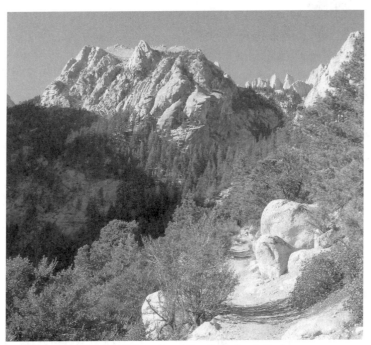

The first view after leaving Whitney Portal: Thor Peak, Crooks Peak, and Keeler Needle

small trickles, which might make for short sections of a muddy trail. Nearby, watch for patches of rose thickets to the side of the trail. In the distance is a collection of pinnacles—the Sierra Crest, just south of Mt. Whitney. Some distance below are the tips of the pine and fir trees growing in the Whitney Portal parking lot. Just before you cross the North Fork of Lone Pine Creek, look for a sign pointing right (northwest) to a use trail: This is the route hikers and climbers take to access the east face of Mt. Whitney and the Mountaineers Route. It also services climbs on 14,088-foot Mt. Russell. You stay on the main trail, crossing the creek on large boulders—or possibly getting your feet wet during the highest flows. On the return trip, you'll appreciate the soft sand underfoot along this stretch of trail.

	North Fork of Lone Pine Creek to the
SECTION **2**	**Lone Pine Lake Junction**
	Distance . . . . 1.9 miles

HINT: Your feet may start to develop blisters along this long stretch of switchbacks. If you feel rubbing, stop promptly to apply moleskin, blister bandages, or sports tape. Stopping for five minutes now will save you time later.

After crossing the North Fork of Lone Pine Creek, sidle around to the head of the canyon, and climb up a long series of switchbacks. They are well-graded, and the trail is sandy with few protruding rocks; if you're doing the one-day hike, this is straightforward walking in the dark. The slope begins under a tree cover of Jeffrey pines and white fir, and then emerges onto a drier slope of chaparral plants. Higher still, some of the larger shrubs disappear, and the slope is covered with a variety of short shrubs and flowers. Near the end of this climb, the trail veers toward Lone Pine Creek, and passes vegetation that requires moister soils—these plants tend to have bigger, thinner leaves. Since this entire stretch of trail is on a single slope with no stream crossings and no junctions, it can feel rather endless; if it is light out, focus on the changes in vegetation and the changing view down-canyon to remind yourself you are indeed making progress. Just past one open patch with a small meadow and a cluster of lodgepole pines, you reach the Lone Pine Creek crossing. A series of raised logs allows you to traverse the broad crossing easily,

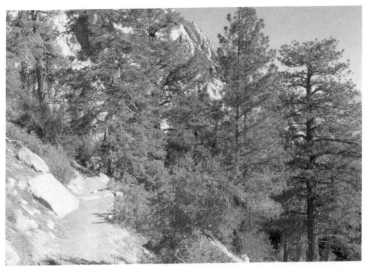

Enjoying scattered Jeffrey Pines on the ascent toward Lone Pine Lake

although during the highest flows you may get wet while approaching these logs. Beyond the stream, you switchback briefly up through lodgepole pine forest and promptly reach the signed Lone Pine Lake junction. Heading left (east) leads to the beautiful round lake, perched on the edge of the long drop-off to Whitney Portal. The Mt. Whitney Trail continues up to the right (southwest).

SECTION 3

Lone Pine Lake junction to Outpost Camp
Distance.............. 1 mile

At the beginning of this section, you enter a sandy flat and pass the sign declaring your entry into the Whitney Zone, where you are required to have a permit. To the south is a blocky talus field flanked by tall, steep cliffs; this is the north face of what is unofficially called Candlelight Peak. Sandier sections mark an area with recurrent rock fall and avalanches.

HINT: Be sure to stop and have a snack as soon as you are hungry. Your body's performance may decrease for the next many hours, if you keep exerting yourself once your muscles start to deplete their glycogen stores.

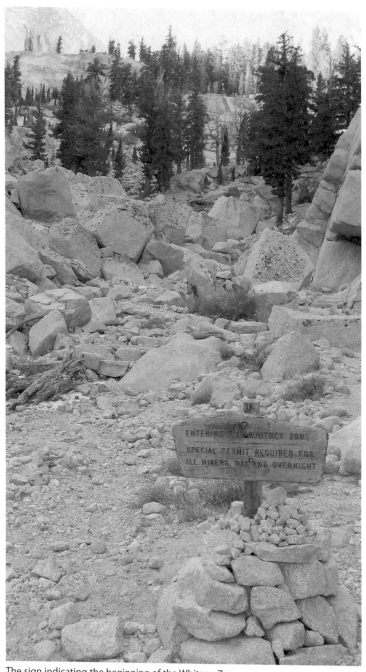

The sign indicating the beginning of the Whitney Zone

Shortly, a series of switchbacks begins, taking you in and out of scattered foxtail pine cover as you ascend. In places, elegant rock walls support the trail. Along this stretch, the lodgepole forests are replaced with the more scattered tree cover characteristic of foxtail pine stands. At the end of the climb, the trail drops slightly into Bighorn Park, a marshy meadow beneath towering cliffs. To your right (north) is the meandering Lone Pine Creek, and to your left are little wet crevices with an enticing collection of small, wetland plants that are rare elsewhere along this trail. At the west end of the meadow is Outpost Camp, the first of the two large campsites along the Mt. Whitney Trail. There are a few small campsites northeast of the trail, but most people choose to pitch their tents southwest of the trail, beneath tall foxtail pines. South of these campsites, Lone Pine Creek cascades over a cliff face in a tumbling waterfall.

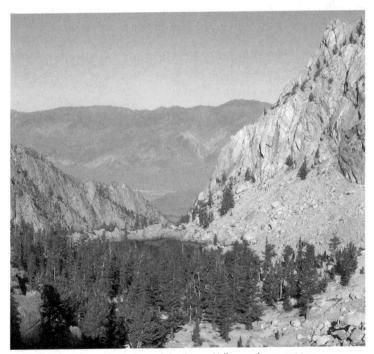

Looking back to Lone Pine Lake and the Owens Valley on the ascent to Bighorn Park and Outpost Camp

SECTION 4

Outpost Camp to Mirror Lake
Distance............... 0.5 mile

HINT: Check your water supply at Outpost Camp or as you cross the Mirror Lake outlet. You should have drunk at least 1.5 quarts by now. If you haven't consumed enough, keep reminding yourself to stop and drink.

For this short stretch of trail, you diverge from Lone Pine Creek, and head slightly north to climb switchbacks along the north wall of the canyon. These south-facing slopes are dry and hot and correspondingly covered with plant species that do well with very little water. The shrub bush chinquapin, with prickly fruit and golden-backed leaves, dominates much of this section, with various colorful flowers growing under-foot. Shortly, the trail intersects the stream drainage and you climb briefly on slabs alongside the creek, before crossing the Mirror Lake outlet on large blocks of rock. To the north is Thor Peak, the large mountain whose steep cliff faces extend all the way to the shores of Mirror Lake. Note that camping is prohibited at Mirror Lake.

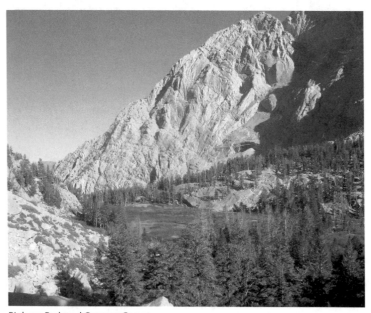

Bighorn Park and Outpost Camp

SECTION 5

Mirror Lake to Trailside Meadow
Distance. . . . . 0.8 mile

Above Mirror Lake, the trail climbs to the top of a small granite ridge and then heads south, back to the main Lone Pine Creek drainage. Scattered campsites exist along this climb, but if you choose to use them, you must carry water up from Mirror Lake, about 0.2 mile below.

HINT: Although the path you are following appears flat compared to the surrounding slopes, the trail continues upward at a good clip— take it easy and pace yourself.

As you ascend, the views down to Lone Pine Lake and Owens Valley are exquisite, especially when early morning light illuminates the granite walls. Along this climb, you pass the last trees, mostly foxtail pines, along with a few stunted whitebark and lodgepole pines. Now in the Alpine Zone, you walk on granite slabs, with a collection of shrubs, herbs, and grasses growing from the base of boulders and out of cracks in the slab. The tall granite walls of the surrounding peaks are suddenly much closer, and to the north, Mirror Lake is

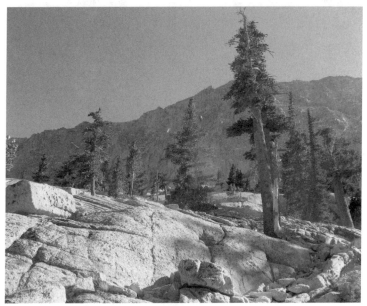

A stand of foxtail pines above Mirror Lake

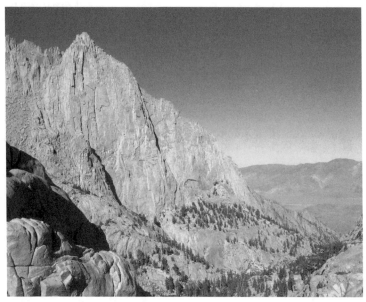

Looking back to Thor Peak and Bighorn Park as you approach Trailside Meadow

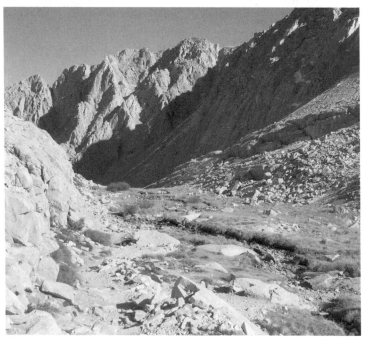

Trailside Meadow

already far below you. The trail mostly follows the crest of a small granite ridge, occasionally dropping into sandy flats that formed along fractures in the rock. Some distance later, you reach Trailside Meadow, an important waypoint: It is almost exactly the halfway point in terms of both distance and elevation. The small meadow, covered with shooting stars, is a refreshing place to take a short break, but camping here is prohibited.

SECTION 6

Trailside Meadow to Trail Camp
Distance .... 1.0 mile

Above Trailside Meadow, the trail makes a couple small switchbacks as it climbs out of the drainage and back up onto slabs. If you look at a topo map, you'll see that you have been following the nose of a small ridge radiating east from Wotans Throne. But shortly, you begin a traverse across a steep slope leading back into the creek drainage. You cross Lone Pine Creek, which is particularly flower-lined at this location, and proceed

HINT: Make sure you have refilled your water bottles before you leave Trail Camp, or fill them at the small spring about a half mile up the switchbacks above Trail Camp. From Trail Camp, you have nearly 9 miles of hiking before you return to water.

up more granite slabs toward Trail Camp. To the south, the skyline from left to right is: Mt. Irvine, appropriately shaped Arc Pass, Mt.

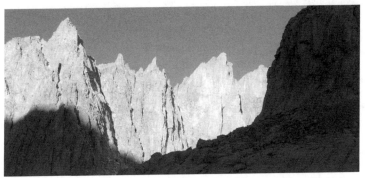

Stopping at Trail Camp to enjoy the first light on the Whitney crest from Mt. Muir north to Crooks Peak

McAdie, and Mt. Marsh, a small summit just beyond Mt. McAdie. Consultation Lake lies below Arc Pass.

Along the last 0.3 mile to Trail Camp, there are many camping options, with water from Lone Pine Creek just a short distance away. Trail Camp itself is a wonderfully scenic campsite and therefore often a zoo of people and tents. There are ample tent sites for everyone, although you can expect to hear the noise of other backpackers and dayhikers long before first light. Since there are no longer toilets tethering you to this specific location, if you want more privacy, search for alternate campsites a bit farther south, or select one of the campsites before you reach Trail Camp.

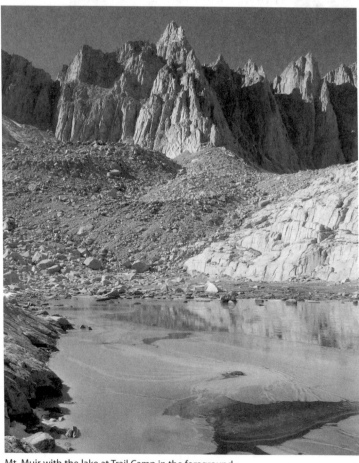

Mt. Muir with the lake at Trail Camp in the foreground

SECTION 7

Trail Camp to Trail Crest
Distance. . . . . 2.2 miles

No one denies that this is a tough stretch of the trail. You are already at 12,000 feet and face a 1600-foot slope with a relentless set of approximately 99 switchbacks—some short, some long, and, luckily, all well-graded. These switchbacks lead to a long talus field via a route that avoids both cliff bands and a large snowfield that can hug the western side of the slope well into the summer. About a third of the way up, you intersect a prominent cliff band where the trail has been blasted into rock. Snow and ice can persist here throughout the summer, so a handrail has been installed for safety. Take a moment to gaze down the steep slab of rock extending below the trail and look up at the colorful and jointed rock

HINT: Many people find it easier to ascend a long slope like this if they can mentally tick off little bits of it as they go. Some possibilities:

- *Count switchbacks.*
- *Carry an altimeter or GPS that tells you the elevation.*
- *Watch the peaks to the north become ever more prominent.*
- *Or, my bizarre favorite when I'm tired: count steps. I just count to 1000 steps over and over again. It keeps my mind focused and I go faster and farther.*

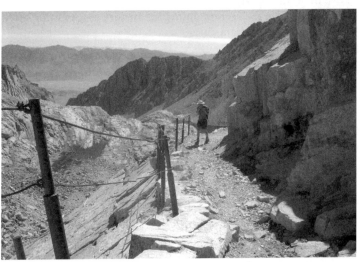

Ascending the stretch of switchbacks blasted into a steep face

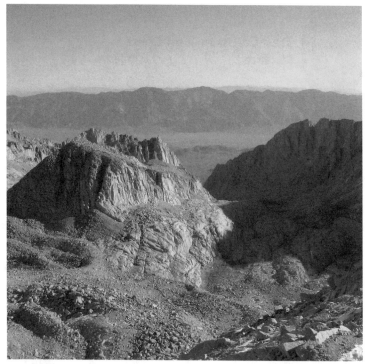

The view down to Wotans Throne and Trail Camp while ascending the 99 switchbacks

above the trail. Above this section, the meager vegetation becomes even sparser. See the section on natural history (pages 14 to 32) to identify some of the plants here.

As you take breathers, stop to look at the mountains. The higher you climb, the more peaks come into view. Mt. Muir, with a sharp summit and tall, steep east arête is the peak nearly due west of Trail Camp, and it dominates the view as you ascend the switchbacks. North of Mt. Muir is the long ridge of pinnacles ending with the flat-topped Mt. Whitney. Mt. Whitney is visible from the lowest switchbacks, but then not again until you are nearly at Trail Crest; Keeler Needle, the next summit south, blocks Mt. Whitney from your view. To the northwest is notably steep Mt. Russell, and to the northeast is the talus field that leads to the summit of Mt. Carillon. The last few switchbacks are longer, and after one final westward traverse, you reach Trail Crest and cross to the west side of the Sierra Crest.

SECTION 8 — Trail Crest to "End of Pinnacles"
Distance............... 1.2 miles

The last miles of the trail to the summit of Mt. Whitney traverse the slope just west of the crest in Sequoia National Park, crossing talus fields and winding among jagged pinnacles. From Trail Crest, you descend briefly but steeply, skirting past a few rock towers and enjoying the view down to the Hitchcock Lakes and up to Mt. Hitchcock. Almost immediately, you reach the junction with the John Muir Trail, where you head right (north). From here to the summit of Mt. Whitney, the Mt. Whitney Trail and the John Muir

HINT: Along this stretch, you are at nearly 14,000 feet. Try to walk so slowly that you don't need to stop more than once every 15 minutes. Just keep thinking, "breathe-step-breathe-step" or even take two breaths per step—just try hard to find that "slow and steady" pace that lets you keep going.

Trail follow the same path. You may see backpacks stashed around this junction, as backpackers arriving from the west generally choose to carry only minimal gear to the summit. Note that the John Muir Trail, which descends the western slope of Mt. Whitney,

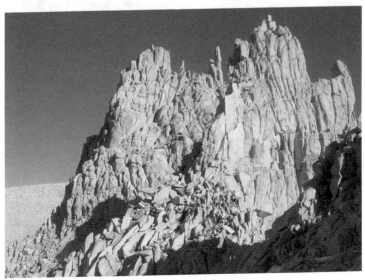

Pinnacles just north of Trail Crest

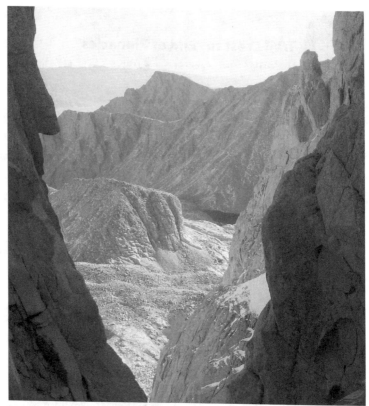

Lone Pine Peak and Wotans Throne (in the foreground) can be viewed through many of the "windows" along the trail

is more pronounced than the Mt. Whitney Trail at this junction, so be sure to take the correct (right-hand) branch. Beyond the junction, you cross a talus field, dotted with bivy sites, some of which are nearly on the Sierra Crest.

At about 13,800 feet, the trail levels off and enters a maze of pinnacles. The slope here has a scalloped appearance, due to the many avalanche chutes that transect it. The many ridges of pinnacles mark the boundary between two avalanche chutes. Between pinnacles, you have open views to the west; in the distance are the dark, jagged Kaweah peaks, while granite slopes dominate the foreground. You repeatedly pass narrow notches, with jaw-dropping views straight down to the east. Near the beginning of this traverse, you may note some rock cairns and well-trod use trails that leave the Mt. Whitney Trail in the direction of 14,012-foot Mt. Muir, a few hundred feet to the east.

CLIMBING MT. MUIR

The summit blocks of Mt. Muir make this a Class 3 climb, indicating scrambling that requires hands and the possibility of falling as much as 20 feet should you slip. However, if you are comfortable with this, the view of Mt. Whitney's summit and the 99 switchbacks are both excellent—and you'll likely have the small summit to yourself. To reach Mt. Muir (only 300 feet away), head east on the small use trail and climb up loose talus until just below the crest. To your left is a steep rock face. Climb up a blocky crack to a 2–foot-wide ledge, and then traverse a few feet to the right into a small gully. Above and left is a 10–foot, blank, low-angle sloping slab, at the top of which are handholds in a small crack. Climb out of the gully onto the slab, which you cross from right to left. Once you are across this, continue up and then right, scrambling between large blocks of rock until you reach a small platform below the summit block. Still on the south side of the summit, climb up this last face to the · top. Note that after the talus section, this entire description encompasses only 50 feet of elevation gain.

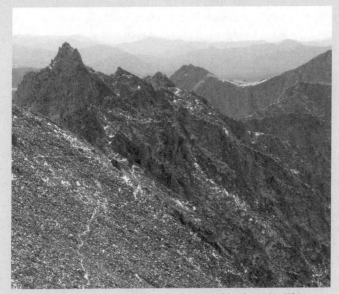

Mt. Muir, viewed from the north on the final switchbacks up Mt. Whitney

"End of Pinnacles" to Mt. Whitney Summit

Distance . . . . 1.0 mile

Leaving the pinnacles behind, you are just 1 mile from the summit. Before you is a large, barren talus field. Large boulders are embedded in sand, with ever smaller numbers of alpine gold and sky pilot growing in sheltered crevices. Traverse across the western face of Crooks Peak (previously named Day Needle) and Keeler Needle, two 14,000-foot points that are too indistinct from Mt. Whitney to be considered true peaks. (Both are straightforward talus climbs from the Mt. Whitney Trail, but they have vertical eastern faces.) Beyond Keeler Needle, the trail bends westward for a stretch, before beginning the final climb to the summit. There are a few half-hearted switchbacks up the last talus field. Nearly all the people heading down will encourage you onward with calls of, "You can't see the summit hut yet, but you're almost there." In fact, due to the summit plateau's very shallow angle, you don't see the summit hut until just minutes before you reach the top. All of a sudden, the views open in every direction. See the labeled panoramic picture on pages 122 to 123 to help you identify the peaks. A large summit register sits by the entrance to the stone hut. Sign your name, then head to the giant boulders a short distance east to take a long, well-deserved break.

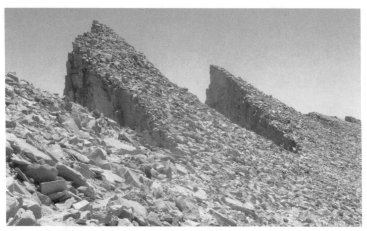

The western slopes of Keeler Needle and Crooks Peak are simply talus piles

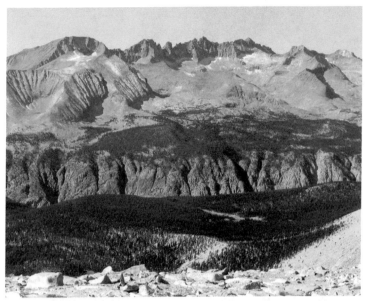

The view west from Mt. Whitney to the Kern Canyon, Kaweah Basin, and the Kaweah peaks

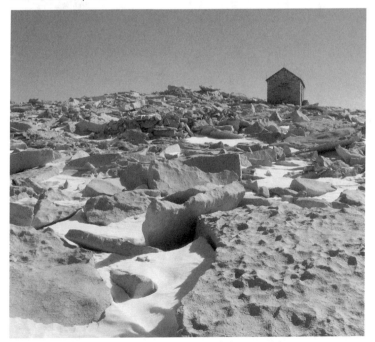

Giant talus blocks dot the summit as you approach the summit hut

PANORAMIC VIEW FROM THE SUMMIT OF MT. WHITNEY

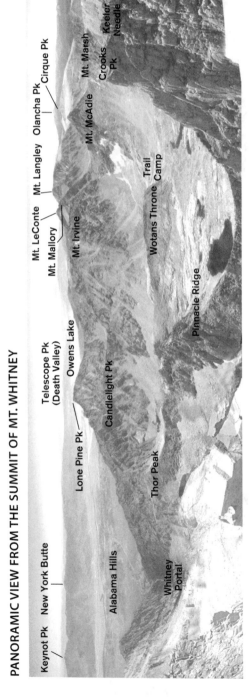

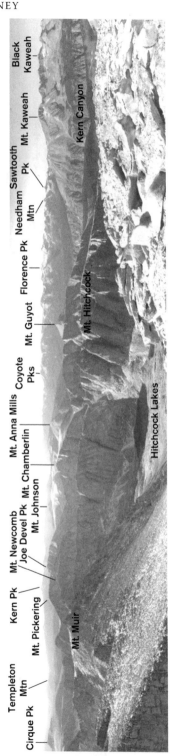

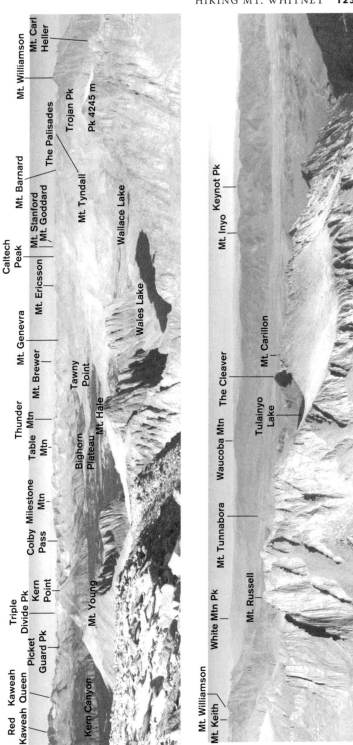

NAMESAKES OF WHITNEY-AREA PEAKS

Much can be learned about the history of this region by learning about the people for whom the peaks have been named. Some peaks bear the names of early explorers, and many others were named by those explorers for the men (yes, they were just about always men) they respected. The spell of astronomy research on the summit around 1900 is obvious. What follows is a short selection; see Peter Browning's *Place Names of the Sierra Nevada* (Wilderness Press, 1991) for information on additional peaks.

Mt. Whitney: Named for Josiah Dwight Whitney, the first California state geologist. For additional information, see page 19.

Mt. Muir: Named for John Muir, the first president of the Sierra Club, an early Sierra explorer, an excellent natural historian, and the person often considered the father of the conservation movement.

Mt. Barnard: Named for Edward Emerson Barnard, an American astronomer in the late 1800s and early 1900s. Among his many discoveries was Jupiter's fifth moon, the last planetary satellite discovered by visual observation.

Crooks Peak: Named for Hulda Hoehn Crooks, a southern California woman who climbed Mt. Whitney nearly each year from age 66 to 91—from 1962 to 1987.

Mt. Hale: Named for George Ellery Hale, an American solar astronomer in the early 1900s. His later career was spent at Caltech, during which time he helped found the school's Palomar Observatory in San Diego County. He passed up many invitations to participate in astronomy research atop Mt. Whitney.

Mt. Carl Heller (Peak 13,211 or 4034 m): Unofficially named for Carl Heller, the founder of the China Lake Mountain Rescue Group in 1958, whose search and rescue efforts saved many lives in the Mt. Whitney region.

Mt. Hitchcock: Named for Charles Henry Hitchcock, a geology professor at Dartmouth from 1868-1908.

Mt. Irvine: Named for Andrew Irvine, who died while ascending Mt. Everest in 1924.

Keeler Needle: Named for James Edward Keeler, an American astronomer who was director of the Lick Observatory on Mt. Hamilton, east of San Jose, California. He was an assistant to astronomer Samuel Langley in 1881.

Mt. Langley: Named for Samuel Pierpont Langley, an American astronomer who made measurements of solar heat from near the summit of Mt. Whitney in 1881.

Mt. Mallory: Named for George Mallory, who died while ascending Mt. Everest in 1924.

Mt. Marsh (the 13,510-foot peak, just southeast of Whitney Pass): Named for Gustave F. Marsh, the Lone Pine resident who built the Mt. Whitney Trail and the Mt. Whitney summit hut. See the book by Doug Thompson and Elizabeth Newbold (Westwind Publishing Company, 2003) for more information

Mt. McAdie: Named for Alexander McAdie, a meteorologist with the San Francisco office of the Weather Bureau who made measurements atop Mt. Whitney in the early 1900s.

Mt. Russell: Named for Israel Cook Russell, an American geologist who was well known for his work around 1890 with the U.S. Geological Survey in Alaska. He was also a professor at both Columbia University and the University of Michigan.

Mt. Young: Named for Charles Augustus Young, an American astronomer in the late 1800s and early 1900s who was a professor at Dartmouth and later Princeton.

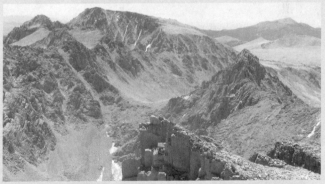

Namesake peaks visible to the south of Mt. Whitney include Mt. Irvine, Mt. Mallory, Mt. Langley, and Mt. McAdie

CELL PHONES AT THE SUMMIT: THE PERSPECTIVE OF A SEQUOIA NATIONAL PARK RANGER

Backcountry rangers have expressed their frustration at the recent trend of people calling 911 from the summit of Mt. Whitney for relatively small injuries. Such calls often result in a helicopter evacuation for a condition that could be remedied on site, allowing the injured person to reach the trailhead himself or with the help of a few extra people.

The rangers' frustration is many-fold: Such rescues are costly, dangerous for the rescuers, and take the "backcountry" out of this backcountry experience. There are extra risks associated with climbing a mountain, and people attempting to summit Mt. Whitney should accept these, rather than looking at their cell phone as an emergency lifeline. Moreover, you should not decide to push your limits just because a helicopter evacuation might be possible.

The Descent

As you retrace your steps to Whitney Portal, keep the following in mind:

- At the junction with the John Muir Trail, the Mt. Whitney Trail heads up to Trail Crest, which means you go south (left).
- Until you are below Outpost Camp, the trail is gravelly and hard underfoot. Thrashing your feet pounding down the upper stretches of the trail is not a wise idea.
- It is especially important to watch you footing on the gravel-covered granite slab between Trail Camp and a bit below Trailside Meadow.
- Keep drinking water and eating food.
- Most accidents occur on the way down a mountain, when you are tired. While you want to get home and minimize hiking after dark, take it easy and take breaks. Also avoid running down the mountain—most injuries, including twisted knees and ankles, occur at the end of the day when you are tired.

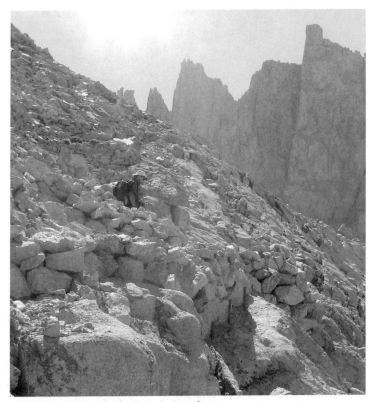

Descending the 99 switchbacks in the late afternoon

STAY ON THE TRAIL

The greatest number of fatalities on Mt. Whitney are due to something that doesn't, at first, seem like a very big risk: heading off-trail. It is tempting for hikers to leave the trail at the snowfield on the east side of Trail Crest and glissade (slide in a controlled manner) down. Unfortunately, many who do this are inexperienced and ill-equipped. No one should ever glissade down a snowfield without an ice axe and preferably a helmet, as well as the knowledge of how to self-arrest. Even if you are carrying this equipment, be aware that this seemingly innocuous snow patch is often icy partway down and many people have lost control, sliding into the rocks below. Be smart and take the switch-backs.

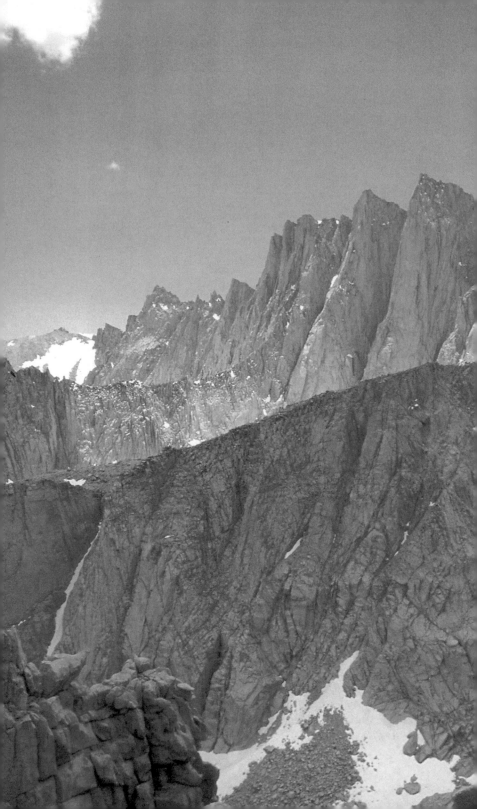

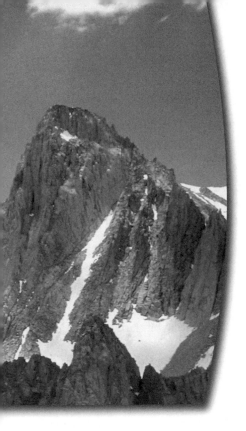

Just a guess, but you may want to celebrate after your hike up Mt. Whitney. The section on Lone Pine and Whitney Portal (see pages 84 to 91), provides a list of restaurants to enjoy. If after a hearty dinner you aren't asleep and decide a dose of alcohol is in order, **Double L Bar** (226 N. Main Street) and **Jake's Saloon** (119 N. Main Street) are two options. (But avoid alcohol the day before you head up the Mt. Whitney Trail, since alcohol and altitude don't mix!) You will probably also want to wander along Main Street in search of some "I climbed Whitney" souvenirs. Suitable T-shirts are available in many stores.

If you have an extra day (or few hours) before heading home, there are a handful of nearby opportunities for sightseeing that do not require much walking—a likely requirement the day after you summited. And for your drive home, stop by the **Interagency Visitor Center** or the **Lone Pine Chamber of Commerce** and pick up a free copy of the Eastern Sierra Roadside Heritage CD produced by the Eastern Sierra Institute for Collaborative Education. On it are 35 minutes of engaging stories about Owens Valley history to make

Opposite and above: The Whitney crest, from Mt. Muir to Mt. Whitney as seen from Russell/Carillon Col

the first part of your drive home pass just a bit faster. (Or you can download the MP3 files from www.roadsideheritage.org.)

The **Beverly and Jim Rodgers Museum of Lone Pine Film History**, located at 701 S. Main Street, is open from 10 AM to 4 PM (closed Tuesday). In addition to an informative 20-minute film recounting the history of films made in the Lone Pine region, the museum is full of props from movies filmed in the area, such as *How the West was Won*, *Gunga Din*, and *Tremors*. Old western and science fiction movies are shown on Thursday and Saturday evenings from late winter through mid October, beginning around 7 PM. They cost $4. If you wish to explore the **Alabama Hills** with a bit of insider knowledge, the Lone Pine Chamber of Commerce website has a map of the Alabama Hills showing where many famous films were shot: www.lonepinechamber.org; go to the site-seeing link.

Manzanar National Historic Site is a bit farther afield. This national historic site is on the location of one of the World War II Japanese war relocation camps, just off Hwy. 395, 7 miles north of Lone Pine. It's open daily in the summer, from 9 AM to 5:30 PM. In addition to a driving loop that takes you past a few outlines of structures from the internment camp, there is a small museum and short introductory film that are worth seeing. See www.nps.gov/manz for additional information.

Recommended Books

Natural History

Blackwell, L. R. *Wildflowers of the Eastern Sierra and Adjoining Mojave Desert and Great Basin.* Edmonton, Canada: Lone Pine Press, 2002.

Gaines, D. *Birds of Yosemite and the East Slope*, Lee Vining, CA: Artemisia Press, 1992.

Hill, M. *Geology of the Sierra Nevada.* Berkeley, CA: University of California Press, 2006.

Jameson, E.W., and H.J. Peeters. *Mammals of California.* Berkeley, CA: University of California Press, 2006.

Weeden, N. *A Sierra Nevada Flora.* Berkeley, CA: Wilderness Press, 1996.

Smith, G. 1978. *Deepest Valley: A Guide to Owens Valley, Its Roadsides and Mountain Trails.* Los Altos, CA: G. Smith Books (Distributed by William Kaufmann), 1978.

Human History

Bowie, W. "Leveling Up Mount Whitney," *Sierra Club Bulletin*, 24:53-57, 1929.

Brewer, W.H., and W.H. Alsup. "Such a Landscape!: A Narrative of the 1864 California Geological Survey Exploration of Yosemite, Sequoia & Kings Canyon From the Diary, Field Notes, Letters & Reports of William Henry Brewer". Yosemite National Park, CA: Yosemite Association, 1999.

Browning, P. *Place Names of the Sierra Nevada: From Abbot to Zumwalt.* Berkeley, CA: Wilderness Press, 1991.

Dyer, H. "The Mt. Whitney Trail," *Sierra Club Bulletin*, 1:1-8, 1893.

Farquhar, F.P. "The Story of Mount Whitney," *Sierra Club Bulletin*, 14:39-53, 1929.

Farquhar, F.P. *History of the Sierra Nevada.* Berkeley, CA: University of California Press, 1965.

King, C. *Mountaineering in the Sierra Nevada.* Lincoln, NE: University of Nebraska Press, 1997.

Le Conte, J.N. "Notes on the King's River and Mt. Whitney Trails (July and August, 1890)," *Sierra Club Bulletin*, 1:93-106, 1894.

Moore, J. G. *Exploring the Highest Sierra.* Palo Alto, CA: Stanford University Press, 2000.

Parsons, M.R. "With the Sierra Club in the Kern Cañon," *Sierra Club Bulletin*, 7:23-32, 1909.

Thompson, D. and E. Newbold. *Mount Whitney: Mountain Lore from the Whitney Store*. El Cajon, CA: Westwind Publishing Company, 2003.

History of Astronomy Research on Mt. Whitney

McAdie, A.G. "Mt. Whitney as a Site for a Meteorological Observatory," *Sierra Club Bulletin*, 5:87-101, 1904.

Osterbrock, D. "To Climb the Highest Mountain: W. W. Cambell's 1909 Mars Expedition to Mount Whitney," *Journal of Historical Astronomy*, 20:77-97, 1989.

Precautions and Considerations

Hackett, P.H., and R.C. Roach. "High-Altitude Illness," *New England Journal of Medicine*, 345:107-114, 2001.

Houston, Charles, et al. *Going Higher: Oxygen, Man, and Mountains*. Seattle, WA: Mountaineers Books 2005.

Wagner, D.R., et al. "Variables Contributing to Acute Mountain Sickness on the Summit of Mt Whitney," *Wilderness and Environmental Medicine*, 17:221-228, 2006.

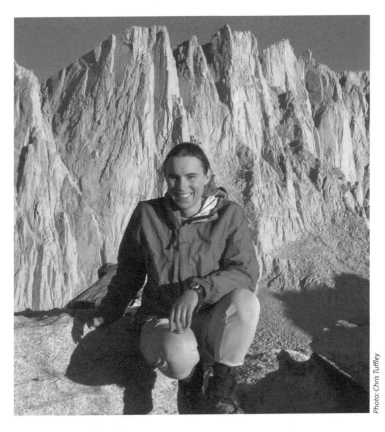

About the Author

Since childhood, Lizzy Wenk has hiked and climbed in the Sierra Nevada with her family. After she started college, she found excuses to spend every summer in the Sierra, with its beguiling landscape, abundant flowers, and near-perfect weather. During those summers, she worked as a research assistant for others and completed her own Ph.D. thesis research on the effects of rock type on alpine plant distribution and physiology. But much of the time, she hikes simply for leisure. Obsessively wanting to explore every bit of the Sierra, she has hiked thousands of on- and off-trail miles and climbed more than 500 peaks in the mountain range. She is especially fond of the steep, rugged peaks in the Whitney region, and she visits the area to hike and climb each year. Lizzy lives with her husband, Douglas, and daughter, Eleanor, in Bishop, California, where she teaches biology at Cerro Coso Community College.

Index

TRAIL NOTES

hot
G...
N...
Kl...
F...
Fire
Sp...
Foot

Gaviota Pk
Middle Fork Cold Sprs (to Camino Cielo)
Upper Oso to Little Pine

Trail Guides and Maps from Wilderness Press

☀ Near Full moon no good

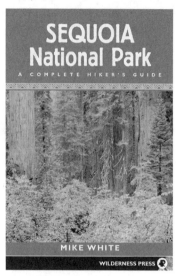

ISBN 978-0-89997-327-2

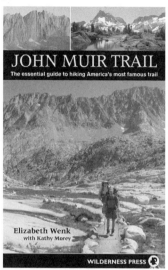

ISBN 978-0-89997-436-1

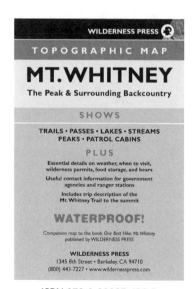

ISBN 978-0-89997-439-2

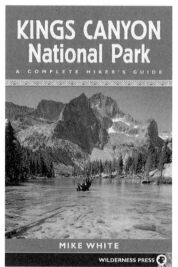

ISBN 978-0-89997-335-7

For ordering information, contact your local bookseller
or Wilderness Press, www.wildernesspress.com

set timer to stop every hour : eat, drink
Electrolytes: fizzie tabs
Sandwiches, energy bars, shot blocks, etc.